CHRIS
BEAT
CANCER

CHRIS BEAT CANCER

A COMPREHENSIVE PLAN FOR HEALING NATURALLY

CHRIS WARK

HAY HOUSE

Carlsbad, California • New York City
London • Sydney • New Delhi

Published in the United Kingdom by:
Hay House UK Ltd, The Sixth Floor, Watson House,
54 Baker Street, London W1U 7BU
Tel: +44 (0)20 3927 7290; Fax: +44 (0)20 3927 7291; www.hayhouse.co.uk

Published in the United States of America by:
Hay House Inc., PO Box 5100, Carlsbad, CA 92018-5100
Tel: (1) 760 431 7695 or (800) 654 5126
Fax: (1) 760 431 6948 or (800) 650 5115; www.hayhouse.com

Published in Australia by:
Hay House Australia Ltd, 18/36 Ralph St, Alexandria NSW 2015
Tel: (61) 2 9669 4299; Fax: (61) 2 9669 4144; www.hayhouse.com.au

Published in India by:
Hay House Publishers India, Muskaan Complex, Plot No.3, B-2,
Vasant Kunj, New Delhi 110 070
Tel: (91) 11 4176 1620; Fax: (91) 11 4176 1630; www.hayhouse.co.in

Indexer: Joan Shapiro • Cover design: theBookDesigners
Interior design: Charles McStravick

A catalogue record for this book is available from the British Library.

Paperback ISBN: 978-1-78817-529-6
E-book ISBN: 978-1-4019-5612-7
Audiobook ISBN: 978-1-4019-5614-1

This book is dedicated to:

MY FELLOW MEMBERS OF THE CANCER CLUB,
who have found themselves on an unexpected journey
and courageously face fear, suffering, and uncertainty
every day while choosing to take massive action
to survive and thrive.

MY PARENTS, DAVID AND CATHARINE WARK,
who love me, encourage me, believe in me,
and have always been there for me. Always.

MY WIFE, MICAH,
who said yes to me, stood by me through everything,
and gave me a beautiful family. You are the love of my life
and my best friend in the whole wide world.

MY DAUGHTERS, MARIN AND MACKENZIE,
who are the greatest joys of my life,
are my proudest accomplishments, and have me
wrapped around their little fingers.

CONTENTS

INTRODUCTION

IT WAS EARLY MORNING and light from a streetlamp was illuminating the edges of the window blinds in our bedroom. Dakota, our blue-eyed husky mix, had her head down, resting on her paws, but her eyes were open. She peered up at me with a look like *What do you think you're doing?*

I was trying to get out of the bedroom without waking up my wife, Micah, who, for all her wonderful qualities, is not a morning person and would no doubt greet being woken up by me with the same level of enthusiasm as a hibernating bear. I gently eased myself out of bed, tiptoed across the bedroom, and slowly slid the closet door open. The wheels squeaked sharply on the track, which was almost ear-piercing in the silence.

I held my breath, grabbed my shoes and clothes, and quickly moved toward the door, motioning for Dakota to follow me. She shook her fur, clinking the tags on her collar, and stampeded across the floor. Micah stirred in her sleep and rolled over.

Outside in the frigid February air, I sucked in a huge breath and held it until I felt the pressure of my heart pumping in my chest and head. Then I let it out, feeling my lungs deflate, and I started to jog down the street. My body felt awkward and uncoordinated, like the tin man. My joints, muscles, and tendons were all still working together, just not very well. The icy, cracked, uneven sidewalk was intimidating and hazardous, but after a minute of hobble-jogging down the hill, things began to loosen up and my confidence grew.

I turned east. The sun was cresting the tree line at the far edge of a parking lot. It was warm on my face, and glorious.

I picked up my pace, stretching my legs with each step until I reached full extension. Then I kicked it into high gear, sprinting toward the light. My legs felt wobbly and dangerous, as if they could fly off my body at any moment. I focused to keep them under control. My heart was pounding, my lungs began to ache, and my legs were burning, but I kept on. As I cut across the parking lot, tears streamed from the corners of my eyes. The wind pounded and whooshed in my ears. I felt alive again. I was running as if my life depended on it. "I'm going to live," I said out loud to myself. "I'm going to live."

Framing cancer as a battle or a fight presents a misunderstanding of the disease. Cancer cells are not alien invaders. Cancer cells are your cells with your DNA. Cancer is not just in you, it *is* you. The presence of cancerous tumors is the result of a breakdown in the normal functioning of your body. Damaged cells mutate and begin to behave abnormally, and the systems designed to identify and eliminate those mutant cells fail, allowing them to rapidly divide and corrupt surrounding tissue with lesions and tumors. Cancer is a condition created by the body that the body can resolve, if given the proper nutrition and care.

Chris Beat Cancer was the name I chose for my blog many years ago because it was catchy, easy to remember, and immediately understood. It is the nickname by which I am identified by readers of said blog as well as my followers on social media, and by default it was the obvious title for this book. But years of research and reflection have changed my perspective. While it is true that cancerous cells need to either die or revert back to normal, I no longer view cancer as an enemy to be beaten or defeated, or a battle to be won or lost. Cancer is not something you fight. It is something you heal.

The purpose of this book is to tell you my story, explain the methods that I and many others have successfully used to heal, and share what I've learned about the power of nutrition and lifestyle medicine as well as the pitfalls of the cancer industry. I've compiled the most important information from my own experience and 14 years of independent research. Much of this information is ignored and/or rejected by the conventional medical community despite mountainous volumes of scientific validation and empirical evidence. As you will see, the research is well documented in this book and freely available for further investigation.

Over the years, I've met people from all over the world who have healed cancer naturally without any medical intervention, and people who have healed cancer after conventional treatments failed and they were sent home to die. These people are not special. They are not superhuman. They are just like you. Thanks to the internet and social media, I have been able to find these people and compare their strategies. I've interviewed many of them, and if you take the time to learn from them and compare the methods they used, you will find common threads that cannot be ignored. The cancer healing revolution is under way. The tipping point is coming.

I'm not a doctor or a scientist. I'm just a guy who chose nutrition and natural, nontoxic therapies over chemo. I was relatively clueless about health and the human body when I was diagnosed, but I devoured as much information as I could find and learned some extraordinary things that changed my life and restored my health. Everything I did, you can do too.

You can change your life. But changing your life often requires a paradigm shift and re-education. We all go through life with various levels of selective ignorance, especially about health and medicine. Ignorance is bliss, but knowledge requires accountability. The reality is that sometimes we just don't want to know certain things because knowing means we will have to make difficult decisions.

Once your eyes are opened, you can't go back. And once you discover that there are many paths you can take to healing, it can be exciting. But it can also create confusion, fear, doubt, and distress.

When my daughters were little, we got a black-and-white kitten we named Cash. When Cash was about three months old, I took him outside to play with us in the front yard. A soon as I stepped outside, he tensed up and dug his claws into my arm. I rubbed his head and stroked his fur, trying to get him to relax, but it wasn't happening.

When I put him down on the grass, he made a beeline for the bushes. And each time I coaxed him out and carried him over to the open grass again, he darted back into the bushes to hide. I realized that Cash was experiencing information overload from all the new sights, sounds, and smells of the outside world. He was instinctively protecting himself from the unknown.

We started taking him outside daily, and after several weeks of cautious exploration, Cash was climbing trees, stalking birds, chasing squirrels, standing up to neighborhood dogs, and napping in the sun, fearless.

The world of health and healing may be completely new territory for you, but don't be afraid. Just step out into the unknown, take it all in, and absorb as much information as you can. You have the power to learn and grow, to deduce the truth, and to discover the right path to restore your life and health.

This information is available to anyone who wants it, but you must be a seeker of knowledge. Anyone who is closed off to new ideas and thinks they know it all, or that doctors know it all, cannot be helped.

The first cancer patient I had the opportunity to share my experience and convictions with was a dear friend named Kathy. I spoke to her at length about why I chose nutrition and natural therapies to build up my body and support healing instead of treatments that would cause more harm. At the end of a long conversation she said, "Chris, I know you're right. I just know you're right. I shouldn't be doing chemo. Deep down I don't feel good about it. Chemo is horrible—it's poisoning my body. Everything you are saying makes so much sense . . ." But she was exhausted physically, mentally, and emotionally and faced an enormous amount of pressure from her family and doctors. In spite of her intuition and instincts, she continued with conventional treatments.

The rest of Kathy's story is typical. The chemotherapy reduced her cancer initially, but within a few months the cancer came back much worse. She was given more aggressive treatments that destroyed her health. In less than a year, she was gone. She left behind a husband and three teenage daughters. Every time I see someone suffer and die after enduring countless rounds of brutal cancer treatments while others are healing, it strengthens my resolve to share this message of hope. True hope. That cancer can be healed.

There is a common misconception that those in the natural health community are anti-science, but this is not the case. I love science. I get excited about scientific research, especially nutritional science, and I will be citing a lot of scientific research in this book. But it is important that we view science in the proper light. Science is not truth. It is an attempt to discover truth. If science were truth, it would always be right. However, not unlike news stories today, there are countless published scientific studies that contradict each other. This has led to a growing mistrust of science in the public eye.

A true scientist is a perpetual truth seeker driven by curiosity and a thirst for knowledge—one who, however passionate about their conclusions and beliefs, maintains an open mind and is always, graciously and with humility, willing to reconsider new evidence; admit that they may be have been wrong; and change their position. Unfortunately, throughout human history the scientific community has been persistently infected with the disease of dogma disguised as skepticism, arrogantly holding fast to established scientific truths of the day, only to be proven false by the discoveries of their successors.

Scientific knowledge is ever evolving, ever expanding, and is rarely ever "settled." As I write this, one of the biggest headlines in the world is that researchers are claiming to have discovered a "new organ" in the human body called the interstitium, and members of the scientific community are now debating whether or not to call it an organ.

When it comes to published science, the people involved matter. Despite the appearance of legitimacy, publishing a scientific study in a peer-reviewed academic journal does not necessarily make it accurate, true, or trustworthy. Scientific research can easily be misunderstood, manipulated, or manufactured. Millions of dollars have been and will be spent funding scientific studies simply to further an agenda, like the infamous studies funded by the tobacco industry that "proved" cigarettes did not cause cancer—until, years later, unbiased scientific studies proved they did.

When confronted with scientific research, before accepting or rejecting its conclusion, at the very least it's important to consider who funded it and who stands to benefit from its findings. Generally speaking, studies conducted by independent researchers without conflicts of interest, with no ties to industry, and with conclusions that cannot be monetized tend to be more trustworthy than, say, drug studies funded by the companies that make the drugs. But there are always exceptions. Bad science can persist for many years, but I do believe that good science, like truth, will win in the end. All of which is to say that I have done my best in this book to highlight compelling scientific evidence, good science from a variety of sources, to help you get closer to the truth and to empower you to make informed decisions—the best decisions for you—to transform your life and restore your health.

INTO THE
JUNGLE

Health is not valued till sickness comes.

— DR. THOMAS FULLER

BY THE TIME I TURNED 26, I had graduated college, married the love of my life, bought 30 rental properties, started a new band with plans to record an album and tour, and just received a call-back to be a potential cast member on a reality show on NBC. Things were going pretty well. As a kid I had always felt I was destined for greatness, and my dreams of proving myself to the world were becoming real. I bounced out of bed every morning thrilled about life. I couldn't wait to see what the future had in store. I felt invincible. Little did I know that five months later all my big plans would take a backseat to survival.

Micah and I met in the 11th grade. She had been dating my friend Russ over the summer, but she and I hadn't met. Micah had a blonde streak in her black hair. She wore Vans. And she had a patch on her backpack of one of my favorite bands, The Cure. I knew she was cool, so I sat by her in history class. It was easy to make her laugh, so much so that the teacher often separated us to opposite sides of the room. A few months later, Micah and Russ broke up, but she and I stayed friends. We ran around in the same social circles and would often see each other on the weekends at local rock and punk shows.

After high school Micah and I both went to the University of Tennessee–Knoxville for our freshman year. Most of our friends were pledging fraternities and sororities, but neither of us were interested in Greek life, so we ended up hanging out a lot. One thing led to another, and by the end of the first semester, we were officially a couple. Six years later, on Valentine's Day, I proposed to her. Three months after that, I graduated from the University of Memphis with a business degree and no job prospects.

Our wedding was set for September. Micah was working full-time and living on her own, and I had moved back in with my parents and was working part-time folding clothes and unlocking fitting rooms at J.Crew. With a wedding date looming, I was feeling the pressure to find a job worthy of my degree and get my act together. After a few interviews, I took a job at a financial planning firm. I had a great mentor, developed some valuable client relationships, and made enough money to get by, but I had a nagging feeling that I was in the wrong profession. I enjoyed helping people, but I wasn't passionate about insurance and investments. It was fun to put on a suit and tie every day, but it kind of felt like a costume.

One day, while sitting in a weekly staff meeting and listening to my boss talk about investment strategies and watching him wipe his leaky eye with his tie for the umpteenth time, I realized there wasn't anyone in the room I aspired to be. I just couldn't see myself staying in a profession I didn't love for the rest of my life only for the money.

I'd been fantasizing about being a professional real estate investor since college, and at the peak of my dissatisfaction in the financial industry, I bought four rental properties in 30 days. It was trial by fire, but I loved everything about it. I loved hunting down deals and finding them before my competitors.

I loved negotiating to get the best price. I loved the renovation process. I loved the idea of building a business that could eventually get me out of the rat race and give me financial freedom. By the end of that year, Micah and I owned 17 rental properties and I quit financial planning to pursue real estate full-time. Thanks to the guidance of a few generous mentors and the infamous bubble-producing federal loan programs, Micah and I were able to buy 31 houses in just two years. I was having a blast and making a name for myself in the Memphis real estate community.

During that time, I started singing and playing guitar in a new band called Arma Secreta (Portuguese for *secret weapon*) with my longtime friend/drummer/now brother-in-law Brad Bean. I was a realist and didn't expect to make much money off my art, and it had been four years since my last serious band. Now, finally, I was playing shows again and Arma Secreta soon picked up speed.

That summer, another good friend named Clay Hurley told me about a new reality show that NBC was casting. He thought it was right up my alley and offered to help me produce an audition tape, so we made one. The casting team liked my audition and asked me to come to Nashville for an on-camera interview. I dusted off my suit and tie, drove to Nashville, and met two of the producers in a hotel room. I felt like the interview went really well until the end, when one of the producers said, "Okay, Chris, now I want you to look directly into the camera and tell Donald Trump why you think you are the next Apprentice."

The question caught me completely off guard because I had no idea what this brand-new show was about, other than that it involved working for real estate tycoon Donald Trump. And I was really uncomfortable talking directly into the camera. So I said something stupid like, "Hi, Donald. I'm a really big fan of your books . . ." The rest is an embarrassing blur. At the time, I was disappointed that I didn't get another callback but not that surprised. And being an *Apprentice* reject turned out to be a blessing in disguise because I had a pesky little problem.

There was a dull aching in my abdomen that would come and go randomly. It was deep and vague. I felt it, but I couldn't quite put my finger on it. There were also sudden twinges of sharp pain that would make me break out in a cold sweat. I remember thinking, *Whoa, what the heck was that? That's not normal . . . hopefully it's nothing.* This eventually progressed to *Uh-oh, there it is again.* Being busy and a stereotypical male not wanting to go to the doctor, I ignored it for many months, thinking it was probably an ulcer and would get better. My body was trying to tell me something, but I wasn't listening.

I've always believed that the human body is designed to heal itself. In this case, I assumed mine eventually would because it always had, but for some reason this time it didn't. The pain gradually got worse. Also, my stool was dark, and sometimes there was a little blood in it. I often woke up in the middle of the night in a cold sweat with aching pain and an urge to go to the bathroom. In the morning, I woke up feeling fine, which is part of the reason I kept putting off seeing a doctor.

Digestive system diseases are especially terrible because they take all the joy out of food. When food becomes a source of pain, you stop eating and your body begins to waste away. At six-feet-two and 150 pounds, I was already thin; I didn't have any extra weight to lose. Most days the pain started an hour or so after dinner, and sometimes I felt it after lunch.

The pain progressed. Eventually, after I spent several nights balled up on the couch after dinner, Micah convinced me to see a doctor. I had blood work and X-rays done, but they couldn't find anything other than slight anemia, and I was misdiagnosed with an ulcer. When the ulcer medicine didn't help, the gastroenterologist decided to do a colonoscopy and an endoscopy (aka upper and lower GI), which means he stuck a camera scope "where the sun don't shine" to have a look around, and then he stuck another one down my throat.

When I regained consciousness, Micah was there beside me. We were in a small room with a curtain for a door, and I was still lying on the gurney. The doctor came in, accompanied by a nurse, and told us he had found a golf ball–sized tumor in my large intestine, and that they were sending a biopsy to the lab to test it for cancer.

I was still groggy from the anesthesia, and my brain was running at half speed. The scene felt like a dream that I didn't understand. And I was too confused to be upset. Micah began sobbing on the shoulder of the nurse, who was the mother of one of our close friends from church. She was a godsend, a tremendous comfort in that moment, and the first of many providential appointments on my cancer journey.

The next day, the phone rang around 7 A.M. It was the doctor calling to tell me I had cancer. He said, "We've got to get you into surgery and get this thing out of you before it spreads. A surgeon will be calling you to schedule surgery as soon as possible." And that was the moment the fear became real and my life came to a grinding halt. It was two days before Christmas. I was 26 years old. And I had cancer.

Of course, my first reaction was *Really? This is my life? I'm the young guy with cancer? Terrific.* The cancer diagnosis made me feel helpless, vulnerable, and weak. Not to mention the fact that I had colorectal cancer, which in my mind might as well be called butt cancer because you know that's what everyone is thinking. And on top of that, this was an old people's disease. I was now the young guy with old people's butt cancer. Spectacular. I had been reduced to an object of pity and sympathy and I didn't like that at all. Humble pie served. Ego destroyed.

When we told our friends and family, they were all shocked. Most were at a loss for words and didn't know how to react. I didn't either.

Before the diagnosis I felt like I was in control, directing the course of my life. But control is an illusion. Sooner or later we all find ourselves face-to-face with circumstances that remind us how fragile life is, and in difficult situations that are beyond our control. This is true desperation.

My wife and I are Christians. We love Jesus. We believe that He is everything He claimed to be. The son of God and the savior of the world. And we believe that the Bible is God's word, eternal truth. At the time of my diagnosis, we were members of a small nondenominational church and I played in the worship band on Sunday mornings.

But my faith was shaken. I couldn't help but think, *God, why is this happening to me? Why am I the one with cancer? I'm one of the good guys, and I'm actually trying do something good with my life!* It begged the classic question "Why do bad things happen to good people?" As I wrestled with this, I remembered Romans 8:28 (NASB):

> And we know that God causes all things to work together for good to those who love God, to those who are called according to His purpose.

I didn't understand why cancer was happening to me, but I knew that God was in control and I chose to believe that He would ultimately work this bad thing out for my good. The next Sunday we stood up in front of our church and told them the news. Nervous and choked up, I quoted Psalms 34:19 (NIV) as a banner over my situation:

> The righteous person may have many troubles, but the LORD delivers him from them all.

The surgeon who was supposed to call me to schedule surgery forgot to call. This turned out to be another blessing. During this time my father mentioned my situation to a co-worker who called in a favor and got me in to see another gastroenterologist for a second opinion. He saw me right away and referred me to an abdominal surgeon who was considered to be the best in Memphis.

I met with the new surgeon, and we scheduled surgery to remove the tumor with a routine colon resection using laparoscopic surgery. The surgeon explained he would only make a few small incisions, just big enough for a camera and his instruments. I asked him how many times he had done this type of surgery. He said, "Hundreds." Good enough. The only other detail I remember from our meeting was how pink and fleshy his hands were, a stark contrast to the pale skin on his arms. I thought, *Man, he must wash his hands a lot.*

There was a heaviness, a sense of sadness and dread that permeated our family Christmas gatherings that year. I tried to act normally, but I was extremely self-conscious. Everyone knew I was sick but most folks didn't bring it up. What was there to say? I was the cancerous elephant in the room.

The day before surgery, I wasn't allowed to eat any solid food except for Jell-O. Micah and I went to a Chinese buffet for lunch after church. She had a plate of delicious-smelling food. I had three different colors of Jell-O. As instructed, I drank a ridiculous amount of a polyethylene glycol solution called GoLYTELY to clean me out that night. It definitely did. Let's just say it was a wild ride and it did not "go lightly."

NEW YEAR'S EVE EVE

On the big day, Micah and I arrived at the hospital bright and early at 7 A.M. to check in for surgery. The woman who admitted me had a note pinned up in her cubicle.

Psalm 23

The Lord is my Shepherd. *That's Relationship!*

I shall not want. *That's Supply!*

He makes me to lie down in green pastures. *That's Rest!*

He leads me beside the still waters. *That's Refreshment!*

He restores my soul. *That's Healing!*

He leads me in the paths of righteousness.
That's Guidance!

For His name sake. *That's Purpose!*

Yea, though I walk through the valley of the
shadow of death . . . *That's Testing!*

I will fear no evil. *That's Protection!*

For You are with me. *That's Faithfulness!*

Your rod and Your staff they comfort me.
That's Discipline!

You prepare a table before me in the presence
of my enemies. *That's Hope!*

You anoint my head with oil. *That's Consecration!*

My cup overflows. *That's Abundance!*

Surely goodness and mercy will follow me
all the days of my life. *That's Blessing!*

And I will dwell in the house of the Lord . . .
That's Security!

Forever. *That's Eternity!*

— AUTHOR UNKNOWN

Her note was such a huge encouragement to me in that moment. I asked her to make a copy of it for me and she did. I still don't know her name, but I thank God for giving us that sweet woman in the admissions office.

After I checked in, they took me to the pre-surgery holding area, where I stripped down, put on a hospital gown, laid on a gurney, and got hooked up to an IV. Doctors, nurses, and hospital staff scuffled about wearing blue covers over their shoes to keep the floors clean. They were just going about their normal, cancer-free lives. I was jealous of them.

Eventually my number came up. Two nurses rolled me down the hall. I was lying flat on my back watching the ceiling lights pass overhead. We turned a corner and I felt the temperature drop.

"They keep the operating rooms colder to prevent the spread of germs," one of the nurses said mechanically. A set of double doors parted to reveal an operating room with six people in full surgical gear: gloves, mask, gown, goggles. All I could see were their eyes, and all eyes were on me. It was creepy. I laughed to myself as they began preparing to sedate me. *These people are all about to see me naked.*

At that moment, I had peace. I knew God was in control. I wasn't afraid. I put my trust in Him, and I was prepared to meet Him if I didn't wake up. The anesthesiologist leaned over and said, "Are you ready?"

"I'm ready."

I took a deep breath and closed my eyes.

After surgery, I woke up in the post-op holding area. My wife and mother-in-law were there with me. I was heavily medicated and tried to speak but could only moan and grunt. I had instructed my wife to bring my video camera to me immediately after surgery so I could document what I might not remember. I somehow managed to turn the camera on and record myself in my weakest, most vulnerable state for a few seconds before turning it off and passing out again. (You can see this at www.chrisbeatcancer.com/surgeryvideo.)

"WAKE UP, SON. WE'VE GOT TO GET YOU ONTO THIS BED"

A series of thoughts slowly bubbled through my pain-medicated brain:

> *Where am I? Hospital room . . . Surgery . . .*
> *Someone's talking to me . . .*

A nurse was trying to get me off the gurney and onto a bed. As I attempted to roll over, I felt as if my guts were being held together by a string and could explode with the slightest flex of my abs. I was in a panic, afraid to move, and the nurse was talking to me like I should just hop from one bed to the other like a kid in a hotel room. With the help of several people, I slowly inched myself onto the bed and passed out again.

The first night was hellish, one of the worst of my life. All I wanted to do was sleep, but I couldn't get any rest because every hour a nurse had to come in and wake me up to do things like take my temperature, check my blood pressure, and turn me over. Thankfully, the nurse assigned to us was an angel. Every time she came into the room, I felt an amazing peaceful presence.

The next day, a nurse changed my bandage. When she pulled it off, I looked down and was surprised to see a six-inch vertical incision going right down the middle of my stomach. The doctor had cut all the way through my abdominal muscles, which explained the sensation I had of my guts exploding. I was simultaneously confused and amused by it.

"Heeeeey, they cut my belly button in half," I said in a dopey slur.

NEW YEAR'S EVE

The surgeon came in and explained that the cancer was worse than they thought. When he put the scope in and looked around, he didn't like what he saw, so he decided to open me up with a large incision. It appeared that the cancer may have spread from the tumor to surrounding lymph nodes. He removed 49 lymph nodes. Four of them tested positive for cancer. I was now stage IIIC. Later that day, an oncologist was brought into my room and introduced to me. I was told that as soon as I recovered from surgery, I would need 9 to 12 months of chemotherapy in order to prevent a recurrence.

At one point during my stay, a med student came in with the attending physician as he made his rounds. He was thin, his skin was pale and yellow, and he had dark circles under his eyes. He looked like a zombie. I thought to myself, *Man, this guy looks worse than I do.*

At this point in my cancer journey, I had accepted that I would do whatever the doctors recommended. I assumed they had my best interest in mind and would take great care of me. But two things happened in the hospital that began to erode my confidence in conventional medicine. The first one was lunch.

The first meal they served me in the hospital after having a third of my large intestine cut out was the worst cafeteria food imaginable: a sloppy joe. Ground up mystery meat stewed in ketchup and slopped onto a burger bun. Don't look for a sloppy joe on a restaurant menu; you won't find it. This mouthwatering delicacy is exclusively available to summer camp goers, soldiers, inmates, and to my surprise, me, the cancer patient.

The heavy pain medication plus the fact that I hadn't eaten in several days did little to soften the blow of this obvious assassination attempt. I asked my wife, "Shouldn't they be giving me something healthier than this? I'm pretty sure this is like the last thing I should be eating right now."

A key indicator that there are no complications with intestinal surgery is a successful bowel movement. And in order to have a bowel movement, you need to eat. Rather than send the sloppy joe back only to have it replaced by something equally terrible like meatloaf, I begrudgingly accepted my fate and ingested the sloppy joe. The next day I had the strangest, scariest bowel movement ever, while standing up in the shower. Good news, everyone: my plumbing is working! Bad news—somebody needs to clean the shower. For the record, that was the first and last time that has ever happened.

After five days and four luxurious nights in the hospital, they gave me permission to go home. The surgeon came by my room to check on me one last time. I was concerned that I might eat the wrong thing and screw the whole surgery up, so I asked him if there were any foods I needed to avoid while my intestines were healing. He replied, "Nah, just don't lift anything heavier than a beer." I chuckled nervously. His dismissive joke and the horrible hospital/prison food were my first indications that the medical establishment did not place much emphasis on nutrition. I was confused by the obvious disconnect between health care and health food. Something didn't add up.

After they released me from the hospital, I went back home to recuperate. Our immediate family and church family were an amazing blessing to us, bringing us meals, praying with us and for us, and helping with anything we needed. I was on heavy pain medication and spent the first week lying on the couch watching movies and sleeping. My friend Brad Stanfill brought me a bunch of videos to watch, including a tape of *Reno 911!* episodes. I hadn't seen it before and I laughed so hard during the first episode that I had to turn it off. I learned an important life lesson that day: abdominal surgery and comedy do not mix.

I stayed on the pain medication for the first week or so but couldn't finish it. I was tired of feeling doped up and instinctively felt like it might be interfering with my healing. Years later, I discovered studies suggesting that opioid-based painkillers like morphine can stimulate the growth and spread of cancer.[1] I also learned that 1 in 10 cancer patients who were prescribed highly addictive opioid painkillers after a surgery like mine become long-term users.[2] My instincts were correct. As I sobered up, I began to think about my life. I wondered what the next year was going to be like for me as a cancer patient. I wondered how much time I had left. I wondered whether I was going to be able to have children. I wondered what my life story would be. Would I live to a ripe old age and see my grandchildren grow up, or would I die young?

I had initially accepted that I would do chemotherapy, but I was developing an internal resistance to the idea. Call it instinct, intuition, or a gut feeling; I didn't have a sense of peace about it. It's important to note that up to this point, I was even more clueless than the typical clueless cancer patient. I had no personal experience with cancer. I had never had any friends or family members diagnosed with cancer, and I knew very little about chemotherapy, except that it was highly toxic and supposedly killed cancer cells. And that it makes you sick, and your hair falls out, and you look like you are dying. The sickest-looking people I had ever seen in my life were cancer patients, but the only two connections I had to cancer were remote. My pastor was a non-Hodgkin's lymphoma survivor, but he had gone through treatment a few years before we met him. And there was another man at our church who had cancer. He was in the printing business and used to play the drums on Sunday mornings before he got sick. People spoke of him often, but I had never met him. I only saw him once, on a Sunday morning. He was bald and his body was emaciated. His clothes hung loosely on his bony frame. His skin was yellow, his eyes were sunken in, and he was obviously weak. He was wearing a surgical mask over his nose and mouth. I couldn't imagine what it was like to be in his condition. He died soon after I saw him, but that one encounter made a dramatic impression on me.

The more I thought about chemotherapy, the less I wanted to do it. The idea of poisoning my way back to health didn't make sense to me, but I was deeply conflicted. So my wife and I prayed about it. I thanked God for everything He had done in my life. I asked Him to heal me, and I asked that if there was another way besides chemotherapy, He would reveal it to me.

Two days later, a book arrived on my doorstep, sent to me by a business acquaintance of my father who lived in Alaska. I started reading the book that day and learned that the author discovered he had colon cancer in 1976. He had seen his mother and many church members suffer and die after undergoing cancer treatment. So he decided to opt out of treatment and radically change his diet and lifestyle. One year after he began juicing and eating a raw-food diet, his cancer was gone. No surgery, no chemotherapy, no radiation. And he was still alive and in excellent health almost 30 years later.

The more I read, the more excited I became. It gave me a new perspective on health, nutrition, cancer, and the cancer treatment industry. His story gave me hope that healing was possible. I thought if he could heal his colon cancer, maybe I could too. That was when I made the decision to take control of my situation, radically change my diet and lifestyle, and do everything I could to support health and healing in my body.

I was so excited and full of faith that I couldn't wait to tell everyone I knew. I called my wife at work and told her I wanted to heal naturally and that I didn't want to do chemo. She thought I had lost my mind. My wife's family is telepathic, so as soon as you tell one person something, everyone knows. Well-meaning family members were soon calling and saying things like, "You have to do what the doctor says. They're using the best therapies available. Don't you think if there was something better they would know about it? Alternative therapies don't work. I know someone who tried that and they died . . ."

This was a new kind of pressure I wasn't expecting. Almost everyone I knew, including my wife, was insisting that I do chemo. Of course, I don't fault them for it. These people loved me and wanted me to live. They were sincerely trying to help but were unknowingly creating a lot more confusion and anxiety. I had prayed and received what I thought was a clear answer, but now everyone was trying to talk me out of it.

So like most cancer patients, in order to appease everyone around me, I reluctantly agreed to go see the oncologist. My appointment was on January 14, 2004. The parking lot to the West Clinic was packed, and so was the waiting room. When Micah and I sat down, I sized up the other cancer patients, curious whether there was anyone else in the cancer club I could relate to. There wasn't. Everyone was two to three times my age. It was surreal. A bunch of old folks and me, the 26-year-old rock dude with shaggy hair and a handlebar mustache. I thought, *God, I don't belong here.*

The TV in the waiting room was on, and one of the guests on the morning show was 89-year-old health and fitness expert Jack LaLanne. Jack came out full of vigor and talked passionately about how our modern diet of processed food was the cause of disease and how a diet of fruits, vegetables, and juicing could transform your health. He said, "If man made it, don't eat it!"

Later they called my name and moved us to a smaller waiting room for additional waiting, and then to a private room where we got to wait some more. Eventually, the oncologist came in. His demeanor was cold and robotic. He gave me what felt like a boilerplate cancer-patient pitch and told me I had a 60 percent chance of living five years if I did chemotherapy, odds that weren't much better than a coin toss. I asked him about a raw-food diet, which I had adopted one week prior, and he told me that I couldn't do it because it would "fight the chemo." I asked him if there were any alternative therapies available. At that moment his demeanor changed; he looked at me dead in the eye and said, "There are none. If you don't do chemotherapy, you are insane."

Instantly I was overcome with fear, and the rest of our appointment was a blur. His tone was arrogant and condescending, and the more he talked the more helpless I felt. I wanted to get up and run out of there but I couldn't. In the midst of his diatribe, he said something that seemed really out of place. He said, "Look, I'm not saying this because I need your business . . ."

When our visit concluded, I felt hypnotized. He had convinced me. And on my way out I made an appointment to have a port installed in a few weeks, the next step before starting chemo. My faith was shattered. I was depressed, discouraged, and afraid. Micah and I sat in her car in the parking lot and cried.

Over the next few weeks I prayed hard and thought hard, desperate for encouragement and direction. I thought about the unhealthy food in the hospital. I thought about chemotherapy making me sicker. I thought about the book that had been sent to me. I thought about Jack LaLanne on TV in the waiting room.

I thought about everything the oncologist had said and how he had treated me. And I realized that God had answered my prayer. I had asked for another way and He had given me one. There were two paths before me, and I had to choose one.

To my left, was a wide, brightly lit road leading to a modern train station where everyone was boarding a beautiful, comfortable, state-of-the-art express train—the chemo train. If I chose that option, I would be surrounded by love and support. People would be cheering me on, raising money, and running races for me. All my needs would be met. But as shiny and attractive as everything seemed to be, I knew that as soon as I got on that train the suffering would begin. And I knew that once I got on, it would be hard to get off. And no one could tell me where I was going. Would they drop me off in Wellville? Or would they kick me off at the end of the line to die, telling me, "There's nothing more we can do"? And if I died, everyone would call me brave, strong, courageous—a fighter, a warrior.

To my right was an overgrown path into the jungle that I had to hack my way through in the dark. There was an official sign posted that said, "Do not enter," and everyone was telling me not to go that way. I knew if I chose that path, no one would understand. I would lose my support, and I would have to go through the journey alone. And if I didn't make it out, if I died on that path, I would be the stubborn fool who refused chemo and my legacy would be reduced to a cautionary tale: "Don't do what Chris did."

Both options were terrifying.

The chemo port installation date loomed larger with each passing day and so did my fear and anxiety. I couldn't shake my internal resistance to it. When the port day finally arrived, I made my choice and was a no-show for the appointment. I naïvely thought that would be the end of it, but the cancer clinic wasn't giving up that easily. They began calling my house and leaving messages trying to get me to reschedule. There were many days when I would come home to a blinking light on the answering machine but avoided pushing play because I didn't want to hear another message. Then they sent me a certified letter that said:

Dear Mr. Wark,

I have been unable to reach you by phone to inform you that your doctor is concerned regarding your missed appointment. Close monitoring of your cancer status is medically necessary to help prevent any life-threatening events from occurring. Please call me to discuss any concerns you might have.

— Robyn

GROUNDHOG DAYS

My first year of cancer was a lot like the movie *Groundhog Day* because every day felt like the same day. Every morning the sun came in through the blinds. I woke up, warm and cozy in bed, feeling good. Then I remembered I had cancer. A wave of fear and cold sweat washed over me. I wondered if I was getting worse or getting better. I got up and became distracted by the demands of the day and forgot about cancer for a little while. But it seemed like every time I turned on the radio or television I heard the word "cancer," and with it came a fresh dose of fear and anxiety.

Despite my fear, I stuck to the plan and continued reading and researching as much as I could about nutrition and natural therapies that might help my body heal. And that's where my mom came in. Enter Catharine Wark. Mom's been into healthy stuff for as long as I can remember. When I was a kid, she bought whole-grain bread instead of white bread, granola instead of Lucky Charms, and natural stir-it-up peanut butter instead of sugary Peter Pan. She froze yogurt and juice to make popsicles, and

I can't remember a time when we didn't have sprouts, kefir, or wheat germ in the fridge.

I never paid much attention to what my mother was reading, but every month there was a new stack of books on her bedside table, and over the years she had amassed an impressive library devoted to health, nutrition, natural medicine, and alternative cancer therapies. Usually people with chronic health problems are the ones driven to research natural methods, but my mom never had any health problems. She was into prevention. In my quest for knowledge, I was continually finding out about more books I wanted to read, only to discover she already had them. For over three decades, she had unknowingly stored up all these books for me. And in the beginning, she was the only person who understood and supported my decision.

During this time, I was also desperate to find other people, real people, who had healed their cancer naturally. The more I looked, the more I found. There was very little information online, but there was an underground network of information that my mom had tapped into through books and videos from alternative cancer doctors, survivors, and researchers. Each new discovery got me more excited about the healing adventure that lay before me.

My mom knew a clinical nutritionist who specialized in holistic health and suggested that I go see him. A few days later a buddy from church brought him up as well. Divine signal received, loud and clear. At that time, the nutritiounist had a modest two-room office in East Memphis. The first time I met him, he was wearing a loose-fitting, beachy button-up shirt, khakis, and clogs. He was a one-man operation, a stark contrast to the multimillion-dollar cancer clinic I'd been in the day before. And his office felt different, peaceful. He was the first person to tell me I was doing the right thing by radically changing my diet to raw food and juicing to support my body's ability to heal. That was a huge validation and a massive confidence booster.

Holistic practitioners are typically not covered by insurance and working with him involved blood tests, saliva tests, urine and stool tests, hair analysis, and lots of supplementation. It wasn't cheap, but it wasn't crazy expensive either. He was looking at the big picture and trying to help me get to the root cause of my disease by correcting nutritional deficiencies, detoxifying my body, and improving my digestion as well as my adrenal and immune function.

My nutritionist referred me to Dr. Roy Page, a surgical oncologist in his 70s who had come out of retirement because he didn't like being retired and wanted to help more people. Dr. Page had spent a lifetime treating cancer patients with destructive and ineffective conventional therapies and in his later years began to integrate nontoxic therapies into his practice. He also supported my decision not to do chemotherapy, which was another powerful confirmation and confidence booster. Dr. Page checked my blood work every month, administered nutritional IV therapy, and ordered a few scans for me along the way.

My team was assembled and my healing plan was in motion, but the first year was tough. There were many days when I was afraid. Like any cancer patient, I was hoping for the best and fearing the worst. The "scanxiety" would build and build until the test results came back. Even though I really liked Dr. Page, I couldn't stand being at the hospital. I felt like a lab rat and couldn't wait to get out. I always left his office on a natural high, skipping down three flights of stairs and bursting outside into the sunlight and fresh air. A few days later, I'd get a call with the results, and Dr. Page was always just as excited as I was. Another good report and a big sigh of relief—thank you, Jesus! Gradually, with each good report came more encouragement, hope, and optimism.

Cancer has a way of cutting a clear dividing line between the important and the unimportant in your life. And I realized that most of the things I cared about before cancer weren't important to me anymore. What mattered to me now was my life and health, taking care of my wife, and starting a family. I really wanted to be a dad, but my cancer diagnosis threatened to postpone fatherhood indefinitely. I was acutely aware of my own mortality and that I might die sometime within the next 10 years. I asked Micah if she would be willing to start a family with me, and she made one of the most courageous decisions of anyone I know. She said yes, knowing she might have to bury me one day and raise our child without me. That's how much she loved me. During my hospital stay, she never left my side. When I wasn't asleep she would squeeze into the bed and watch marathons of *MythBusters* and *American Chopper* with me.

We found out Micah was pregnant four months after my diagnosis, but when we told family members the reactions were mixed. Some were excited and others were concerned about the timing. But good timing or not, this baby was coming. One year after my cancer diagnosis, I was back in the hospital. But this time I was holding our beautiful little baby girl in my arms. We named her Marin Elizabeth, and I now had someone else to live for.

In the years that followed, I did what most cancer survivors do. I distanced myself from cancer. I didn't want to think about it or talk about it. I just wanted to get back to living a normal life. I continued investing in real estate, flipping houses, and doing custom home renovations. Our second daughter, Mackenzie Rae, was born in June 2008, a week after I turned 31. My band, Arma Secreta, recorded and released two records, *A Century's Remains* and *Dependent Lividity*, and played hundreds of shows in the Midwest and on the East Coast.

Eventually my story got around and people were constantly asking me about my health—why I didn't do chemo and what I did instead—and I realized that I had something important to share with the world.

Seven years after my diagnosis, I started a blog called *Chris Beat Cancer* to give people inspiration, encouragement, and resources on healing and preventing cancer with nutrition and natural, nontoxic therapies. I created the site to be what I wished had existed for me back when I was lost and confused. I knew there were people out there just like me, with a fresh cancer diagnosis looking for answers. As the blog gained exposure, messages began to come in from people all over the world who had healed cancer without conventional treatment or after conventional treatment had failed them, including stage IV cancers. I began interviewing them and sharing their stories on chrisbeatcancer.com, and I realized how important it was to show the world that cancer can be healed and that real people are doing it.

My decision to "go public" with a blog completely changed the course of my life. I've had the opportunity tell my story many times on radio, television, and film. I was featured in the award-winning documentary film *The C Word* and on *The Truth About Cancer* series. I've been a part of online summits like The Food Revolution and Food Matters, and I've had the privilege of traveling to and speaking in places I never dreamed of, including London, Moscow, and even Cambodia. Sharing information that can help people heal and prevent cancer as well as navigate cancer treatment has become my life's work.

The five-year relative survival rate for stage IIIC colon cancer is 53 percent.[3] Young adult patients (under 40) have a 28 percent higher risk of cancer progressing and spreading during a one-year follow-up, and are 30 percent more likely to die from cancer.[4,5] According to the National Cancer Institute, stage III colon cancer patients with one to three involved lymph nodes have significantly better survival than those with four or more involved nodes.[6,7] I had four. Furthermore, a meta-analysis of studies found that colon cancer patients with tumors on the left side have better survival rates.[8,9] Mine was on the right.

Even though the odds of long-term survival were stacked against me, this year I celebrate my 15-year "cancerversary." I am so thankful to be alive. God is good. I put my trust in Him, and He led me in the path of healing.

I want to be very clear that I am not "lucky" or special. I am just a regular guy who listened to his instincts, stepped out in faith, and took massive action to help his body heal. I eliminated everything in my life that may have contributed to my disease, and changed the internal terrain of my body—making it a place where cancer could not thrive. What I did, I believe anyone can do, including you.

I'm going to show you what I've learned in the last 15 years of researching nutritional science, the cancer industry, and people who have healed cancer.

You will discover where conventional medicine went wrong, why the cancer industry has failed to win the war on cancer, and how you can avoid the common perils and pitfalls of cancer treatment. You will also learn the exact steps I took to radically change my life and heal. These actionable diet and lifestyle strategies are not unique to my journey. They are common threads among everyone I know who has healed cancer. Wherever you are in your health journey, whether you are trying to heal or prevent cancer, these are strategies you can implement in your life right now. So let's begin.

SURVIVAL OF
THE SICKEST

The problem is not to find the answer;
it's to face the answer.

— TERENCE MCKENNA

IN 2010, RESEARCH SCIENTISTS Professor Rosalie David and Professor Michael Zimmerman published a study on the origins of cancer. They examined nearly a thousand mummies from ancient Egypt and South America, as well as fossils and ancient medical texts, looking for evidence of cancer in our ancestors. They only found five cases of tumors out of a thousand mummies, and only one of those tumors was thought to be malignant.[1]

The earliest scientific literature describing what we now call cancer is dated thousands of years later. Notes dating back to the 1600s described operations for breast and other cancers. In 1761, snuff users were documented to have nasal cancer. Chimney sweeps were developing scrotal cancer in 1775. Hodgkin's disease was first noted in 1832. Some have asserted that the discovery of cancer in a few mummies dispels the notion that cancer is a "man-made disease," but that's not what the expression implies. The incidence of cancer has exploded as a result of the significant changes humanity has made to the world in which we live, and the way we live in it.

Perhaps the most fundamentally misunderstood aspect of cancer is that it is not a singular disease. The term "cancer" is a catch-all term for a broad array of unique diseases in the body that can eventually lead to uncontrolled cell growth. There are over 200 different types of cancer, which is why there will never be a singular "cure" for cancer.

THE PLAGUE OF PROGRESS

Even though cancer is not a singular disease, there is a singular point in history where the incidence of cancer began to snowball: the Industrial Revolution. Factories were built to mass-produce everything: fossil fuels, building materials, textiles, furniture, food, chemicals, and all sorts of exciting innovations. The Industrial Revolution paved the way for all the modern conveniences we enjoy today, including electricity, cars, planes, computers, and smartphones, but it also produced an unfortunate by-product: industrial pollution. Many of the chemicals used in the production of modern goods are highly toxic, and many production processes create toxic waste by-products that have polluted our air, water, soil, food—and our bodies. It's estimated that as many as one in five cancers are caused by environmental pollution.[2]

Air pollution from planes, trains, and motor vehicles, as well as home heating and industrial exhaust, is linked to all sorts of chronic diseases. Exhaust from diesel engines is known to cause lung cancer.[3] Even if you don't breathe polluted air, the pollution can still find its way into your body. Coal-burning power plants spew mercury-laden exhaust fumes into the air, which eventually end up in our water supply and in the flesh of fish we eat, especially in predators like tuna. For decades, factories have quietly polluted our environment with toxic cancer-causing waste like polychlorinated biphenyl (PCB) and hexavalent chromium (think *Erin Brockovich*).

Geographical areas where cancer rates are particularly high due to pollution are known as cancer clusters, and these clusters are usually industrial areas. In 2013 researchers at Emory University found an increased risk of non-Hodgkin's lymphoma among people who lived near factories that released benzene into the environment.[4] Benzene is used in the production of plastics, nylons, resins, and other materials such as lubricants, dyes, cleaners, and pesticides. The closer the people lived to benzene-releasing factories, the higher their risk.

In the United States, there are over 80,000 chemicals registered with the Environmental Protection Agency (EPA) for use in food production, cosmetics, prescription drugs, household cleaners, lawn care, agriculture, and more. These chemicals are in nearly every man-made product you buy, including makeup, plastics, paints, stains, varnishes, fabric dyes, and flame retardants. Full safety test data is available for a small percentage of these chemicals, but over half of them have no safety testing data at all.

Many of these chemicals are considered to be harmless in small amounts, but this is based on the assumption that everyone will only be exposed in small, isolated doses. What isn't taken into account is the synergistic toxicity created by exposure to thousands of these chemicals over one's lifetime.

In 2015, a task force of 174 scientists from 28 countries identified 50 common chemicals considered to be harmless at low doses but that could become carcinogenic when combined with other "harmless" chemicals. Some of the chemicals identified include triclosan in antibacterial soap; phthalates in plastics; titanium dioxide used in sunscreen; and acrylamide, which is found in french fries, coffee, some cereals, bread crust, and roasted nuts. According to cancer biologist and study author Dr. Hemad Yasaei of Brunel University in London, "This research backs up the idea that chemicals not considered harmful by themselves are combining and accumulating in our bodies to trigger cancer and might lie behind the global cancer epidemic we are witnessing."[5]

When you consider all of the chemicals in our environment, as well as those added to our food and in products we use every day, it can be a bit overwhelming. We are swimming in a toxic soup with a risk that is impossible to calculate.

THE POWER OF YOUR CHOICES

"We're all going to die sometime" is a popular bad habit justifier employed by people who don't think that their diet and lifestyle choices matter. But your choices do matter. It is now estimated that 70 percent of premature deaths from preventable diseases in the United States are attributed to three factors: poor nutrition, lack of physical activity, and tobacco use.[6,7] And when it comes to cancer, a recent study published in *Nature* estimated that as many as 70 to 90 percent of cancers are caused by diet, lifestyle, and environmental factors.[8]

It should be noted that before death come years of chronic disease and disability. According to a RAND Corporation study, 60 percent of Americans have at least one chronic condition and 40 percent have multiple chronic conditions. Nearly 150 million Americans are living with at least one chronic condition; around 100 million of us have more than one. And nearly 30 million Americans are living with five chronic conditions or more.[9] Our top killer chronic diseases—cardiovascular disease, cancer, and type 2 diabetes—are for the most part not genetic. They are not caused by bad luck or bad genes. They are directly connected to our choices. Your choices have the power to create health or disease in your body.

ONCE UPON A TIME IN THE WEST

Before we continue, I would like to clarify some terms you will see throughout this book. The Industrial Revolution is a product of Western civilization, which is why industrialized countries are also referred to as Western nations. The diet consumed by industrialized Western nations is known as the Western diet, and the chronic noninfectious diseases common to these nations—like heart disease, diabetes, and many cancers—are known as Western diseases or diseases of affluence. The Western diet is characterized as being high in animal products, especially red meat and dairy; high in refined sugar, saturated fat, junk food, and processed food; and low in fresh fruits, vegetables, legumes, nuts, seeds, and whole grains. The Western diet has its roots in the United States but in the last half century has been exported around the world, and today it has little to do with geography. For example, most European countries are located in the Eastern hemisphere but are considered to be Western nations eating a Western diet and getting Western diseases.

EVERYBODY THINKS THEY ARE HEALTHY

Fewer than 3 percent of Americans are considered to be living a healthy lifestyle, which is made up of four factors: eating five servings of fruits and vegetables daily, getting regular daily exercise, not being overweight, and not smoking.[10,11]

Thanks to a lifetime of food industry marketing, most of us have been conditioned to believe that we eat pretty healthy. The surprising reality is that only about 10 percent of Americans are eating the recommended amount of fruit and vegetables per day.[12] Americans eat an average of 1.7 servings of vegetables per day. Only 2 percent of the American diet is whole fruits, and 3 percent of it is vegetables other than potatoes. Another 3 percent of it is beans and nuts, and 4 percent of it is whole grains like oats, barley, whole wheat, and brown rice.[13,14,15]

Nineteen percent of the American diet consists of foods made from highly processed grains like white flour and corn starch, such as white bread, bagels, muffins, and tortilla chips. Seventeen percent comes from added sugars in soda, candy, and processed food, and 23 percent comes from added fats like butter and margarine, as well as shortening and oils from corn, canola, and soybeans, which are widely used in processed and fried foods and are predominantly made from genetically modified crops.

The remaining 26 percent of the American diet consists of meat, dairy, and eggs, the health benefits of which are widely (and hotly) debated. If you consider animal foods to be healthy, the typical American diet might be about 38 percent healthy and 62 percent unhealthy. If you view animal products as unhealthy, the average American's diet is around 12 percent healthy and 88 percent unhealthy. This doesn't take into account the difference between organic, pasture-raised animal products and those that come from commercial factory farms, which divides the debate further. Either way, both positions offer insight as to why the Western diet has led to industrialized nations suffering from chronic Western diseases in epidemic proportions.

A study published in 2018 offered key insight into how highly processed food may cause inflammation in the body and make the immune system more aggressive over time. Mice fed a high-calorie, high-fat, high-sugar, Western fast-food diet for a month were found to have high levels of immune system activity and inflammation in their bodies, surprisingly similar to how the body responds to a bacterial infection. After the mice were put back on their normal diet for four weeks, the inflammation went away, but some of the genetic switches in their immune cells stayed on, keeping their immune systems on high alert with a tendency to overreact to small stimuli with stronger inflammatory responses.[16] An overly aggressive immune system triggered by the Western diet could be the missing link behind why so many people suffer from chronic inflammation, which makes your body a breeding ground for cancer.

Another 2018 study found that every 10 percent increase in consumption of ultra-processed foods increases your cancer risk by 12 percent.[17] Ultra-processed foods include sugary drinks, processed baked goods, sugary cereals, salty snack foods, reconstituted meat products, and ready meals like instant noodles and soups and TV dinners. The scary reality is that more than half the foods Americans and U.K. citizens eat is ultra-processed, which gives us roughly a 60 percent increase in cancer risk compared to people around the world who don't eat a Western diet loaded with ultra-processed food. Even just one sugary soft drink per day has been linked to an increase in risk of 11 different cancers, including breast, kidney, liver, colorectal, and pancreatic cancer.[18]

OUR LEADING CAUSES OF DEATH

The Western diet causes Western diseases like heart disease, cancer, and diabetes. Heart disease is the leading cause of disease death in the U.S., killing about 595,000 people annually. Cancer is close behind, killing about 580,000 people per year. Cancer is already the leading cause of death in 22 states and is expected to take the number one spot in the U.S. in the coming years. The vast majority of incidences of these killer diseases are not caused by bad luck or bad genes. They are the direct result of our daily diet and lifestyle choices compounded over time. Lung cancer is the number one cancer killer for men and women, and smoking causes roughly 90 percent of lung cancers and at least 30 percent of other cancers, including digestive cancers, head and neck cancers, ovarian cancer, and leukemia.

Smoking also increases your risk for liver, cervical, breast, prostate, and skin cancer because when you smoke, carcinogenic toxins circulate and pollute your entire body. Along with causing cardiovascular disease, smoking is the number one cause of cancer and cancer death. The good news is that you can reduce your risk of lung cancer by roughly 90 percent by not smoking.

Like smoking, alcohol is also classified as a Group 1 carcinogen. Alcohol is responsible for over 5 percent of new cancer cases each year and nearly 6 percent of cancer deaths worldwide. The highest cancer risk is in heavy long-term drinkers who also smoke, but the latest research indicates even just one drink per day for women and two drinks per day for men increases risk over one's lifetime.[19]

LADIES AND GENTLEMEN, WE ARE FAT

We have an unlimited supply of food, and our calorie consumption has increased significantly over time. According to the USDA, the average American ate 3,400 calories per day in 1909. Today the average American eats roughly 4,000 calories per day, 600 more calories per day than we were eating 100 years ago. Two-thirds of American adults and nearly 30 percent of boys and girls under age 20 are overweight or obese. Millennials are on track to be the fattest generation in recorded human history by the time they reach middle age.[20] According to recent estimates, half of Americans don't get enough physical activity, and over one-third of us are actually classified as "physically inactive,"[21] mostly the obese third. Obesity kills roughly 110,000 Americans each year; it is the second leading cause of cancer behind smoking, and it is quickly approaching the number one spot.

Obesity causes over 600,000 cancers each year, roughly 40 percent of all cancers.[22] Excess body weight contributes to insulin resistance, abnormal hormone levels, chronic inflammation, decreased immune function, and significantly increases your risk for 13 different cancers, including colorectal, endometrial, ovarian, pancreatic, thyroid, and postmenopausal breast cancers.[23]

For decades, doctors have advised patients to maintain a healthy weight and keep their body mass index (BMI) in a normal range (between 18.5 and 25) in order to reduce their risk of obesity-related diseases and cancers. But a normal BMI doesn't necessarily mean health when chronic disease is the norm. Surprising new research published in 2018 revealed that having a high percentage of body fat can double a woman's risk for invasive estrogen-positive breast cancer even if she has a normal weight and a normal BMI.[24] Visceral fat, also known as belly fat, which is deposited around abdominal organs such as the liver, pancreas, and intestines, may be the biggest troublemaker. Belly fat produces a protein called fibroblast growth factor-2 (FGF2), which has been demonstrated to drive certain vulnerable skin and mammary cells to transform into cancerous cells.[25]

Excess body fat is primarily caused by poor diet and lifestyle choices, specifically a high-calorie diet with too much white sugar, white flour, refined oils, and animal foods and a lack of exercise.

Our top two causes of cancer come from what we are putting in our mouths—cigarettes and unhealthy food.

AN EXPLOSION OF INACTIVITY

Along with our unhealthy diets, modern conveniences have led to a sedentary lifestyle for modern earthlings compared to our ancestors, who walked everywhere and did physical work every day. They grew crops, hunted for food, raised livestock, ran from tigers, climbed trees, built shelter, danced around the fire, and crafted their tools, clothes, and furniture by hand. They were strong, fit, and rarely overweight, with the exception of the rich.

Now let's compare that to a typical day for someone in a first-world country. After lying down all night, we get up and get ready for the day. We bathe and get dressed. Then we sit down to eat breakfast. Then we sit in a car, bus, or train that carries us to work. Once at work, we sit at our desk to do said work. A few hours later, we get up to eat lunch. Then we find somewhere to sit down and eat it. Some of us eat lunch right there at our desks without getting up at all. After lunch, we do some more sitting at work. Then we have a seat in a car, bus, or train to travel home from work. When we get home, we have a nice sit-down dinner followed by some sitting on the couch or in bed to watch TV and/or surf the internet until bedtime, when we lie down for the night.

Granted, not everyone is *that* sedentary, but many of us are. The bottom line is that we just aren't moving our bottoms enough. On average, we Americans spend roughly 15.5 of our 16 to 17 waking hours each day sitting. Prolonged sitting significantly increases your risk of heart disease, diabetes, and cancer. According to epidemiologist Dr. Christine Friedenreich, physical inactivity is linked to as many as 49,000 cases of breast cancer, 43,000 cases of colon cancer, 37,000 cases of lung cancer, 30,000 cases of prostate cancer, 12,000 cases of endometrial cancer, and 1,800 cases of ovarian cancer. All totaled, prolonged sitting is estimated to contribute to 173,000 cases of cancer per year. Three to six hours per week (30 to 60 minutes per day) of moderate to vigorous exercise, ranging from walking to intense aerobic exercise, has been linked in numerous studies to a 20 to 40 percent reduction in cancer risk for 13 types of cancer.[26,27]

THE FOOD FACTOR

Over the last century, the quality of our food and the quantity that we are eating have changed drastically. Our overall carbohydrate intake has come down about 4 percent, but the types of carbohydrates we eat are very different. In the early 1900s, most of our carbohydrates were from whole foods like grains, beans, and potatoes. Today most of our carbohydrates are from refined foods like white flour, sugar, corn syrup, sugary drinks, potato chips, and french fries. We're also eating about 20 percent more animal protein than we were in 1909 and 60 percent more fat, primarily from oils.

Polyunsaturated fats in our diet, from corn, soybean, and sunflower oils and fatty fish are up 340 percent. Monounsaturated fats from olive, peanut, safflower, and sesame oils are up 70 percent. And saturated fat, mainly from butter and lard in animal foods, is up 20 percent. We are also eating roughly 10 percent more cholesterol. All totaled, our fat consumption has increased 60 percent from oils and animal foods in the last 100 years.[28]

Fresh food has been replaced by fast food. A hundred years ago, giant supermarkets and restaurant chains didn't exist, and it was common for a household to keep a vegetable garden and livestock for food. Today this practice is a rarity in the Western world, and the food that most people assume is healthy has been hijacked.

Food manufacturers strip food of its nutritional value and then add unnatural chemical ingredients, including artificial flavors, colors, additives, preservatives, and texture enhancers, as well as refined sugar and salt, hydrogenated oils, and trans fats.

The food industry has replaced natural ingredients with artificial ones to increase the profit margin and shelf life of their products. Simply put, artificial strawberry flavor is much cheaper than real strawberries.

Caramel coloring, produced with ammonia, is one of the most widely used food colorings in the world. It is used in colas, beer, sauces, and more, and it has been identified as a carcinogen. The state of California requires food manufacturers to put a warning label on food that contains more than 29 micrograms of caramel coloring.[29]

Agricultural giants are growing produce with toxic chemical fertilizers, pesticides, and herbicides. Many fruits and vegetables are picked before they are ripe and then artificially ripened with ethylene gas. These GMOs (genetically modified organisms) are genetically engineered with DNA from bacteria, viruses, or other plants and animals to withstand toxic herbicides like glyphosate (found in Roundup) and to produce their own insecticide.

Numerous studies have shown that GMO foods can be toxic or allergenic, and hazardous to people and animals that eat them, and many developed nations do not consider GMOs to be safe. Over 60 countries, including Australia, Japan, and the European Union, have significant restrictions and/or outright bans on the production and sale of GMOs. Unfortunately, in the U.S. it's a different story. U.S.-grown alfalfa, canola, corn, papaya, soy, sugar beets, zucchini, and yellow summer squash are predominantly genetically modified.

THE MYSTERY MEAT MACHINE

The vast majority of our meat today comes from factory farms where livestock are fed grain-based feed, injected with growth hormones, and given antibiotics to help prevent sickness while living in cramped, unsanitary conditions.

Commercial dairy cows are injected with recombinant bovine growth hormone (rBGH) under the brand name Posilac. This is a genetically engineered hormone introduced by Monsanto in 1995 that increases milk production in dairy cows by about 20 percent. rBGH also increases insulin-like growth factor 1 (IGF-1) in cow's milk. Elevated levels of IGF-1 can promote cancer in humans, specifically endometrial, prostate, breast, pancreatic, and colon cancer.[30] A European Commission report stated that "avoidance of rBGH dairy products in favor of natural products would be the most practical and immediate dietary intervention to . . . (achieve) the goal of preventing cancer."[31] rBGH has been banned in all 25 European Union countries, as well as in Canada, Japan, Australia, and New Zealand, but not the United States.

BREAD IS DEAD

A major source of calories in the Western diet comes from white flour and white bread, but nutritionally speaking, bread—specifically white bread—is dead. Whole organic grains, including whole wheat, are health-promoting staple foods consumed by the longest-living people on earth, and contain phytonutrients known to have protective effects against several types of cancer, especially colon cancer.[32] But when whole wheat is refined into white flour, it is stripped of 25 naturally occurring nutrients and then "enriched" by adding back only 5 isolated nutrients that were removed. Then chemical additives and preservatives are added to make the bread fluffier and increase its shelf life.

White flour is an unhealthy food, and we're eating it at nearly every meal. We're eating cereal, toast, muffins, biscuits, bagels, pancakes, and waffles for breakfast, and we're eating sandwich bread, burger buns, tortillas, pizza, pasta, and rolls for lunch and dinner. And let's not forget snacks and desserts like crackers, cookies, cakes, and pies. White flour converts to sugar in your bloodstream and gives you energy, which is good. But unlike whole-food carbohydrates (fruits, veggies, and whole grains), it lacks beneficial phytonutrients and antioxidants, which neutralize the toxic free radical by-products of cell metabolism. White flour and white sugar are empty calories, and a diet rich in empty calories will eventually make you fat and sick.

To make matters worse, conventionally grown wheat is sprayed with glyphosate (the active ingredient in Roundup) to control weeds and help dry it out 7 to 10 days before harvest. A 2009 article in the journal *Toxicology* cited evidence that glyphosate-based herbicides are endocrine disrupters at trace amounts of just 0.5 parts per million (ppm) and are liver toxic at 5 ppm in humans.[33] Gluten-free foods are all the rage these days, but gluten may not be the real problem for many folks. A 2013 article in *Interdisciplinary Toxicology* reported that the incidence of gluten intolerance, celiac disease, and irritable bowel syndrome has risen in direct proportion to the increased spraying of glyphosate on conventionally grown grains including wheat, rice, seeds, beans, peas, sugar cane, sweet potatoes, and sugar beets.[34] In 2015 the World Health Organization International Agency for Research on Cancer classified glyphosate as "probably carcinogenic to humans." Glyphosate is not only sprayed on genetically modified "Roundup-ready" corn, canola, and soybeans, but it is also sprayed on many types of conventionally grown non-GMO grains and vegetables to dry them out before harvest, including wheat, millet, flax, rye, buckwheat, barley, oats, beans, peas, lentils, corn, potatoes, and more.

MERCURY RISING

Mercury is the only naturally liquid metal on earth and is also classified as a "heavy metal." But despite its unique awesomeness, mercury is also a neurotoxin that has been linked to immune system suppression and a host of physical problems including brain damage, autism, Alzheimer's, amyotrophic lateral sclerosis, multiple sclerosis, cancer, and other chronic diseases. Very small amounts of mercury can damage the brain, nervous system, heart, lungs, liver, kidneys, thyroid, pituitary and adrenal glands, blood cells, enzymes, and hormones.

Mercury is a naturally occurring element that is all around us in our environment, but industrial pollution has doubled that amount. The majority of mercury pollution is spewed into the air by coal-fired power plants. From there it finds its way into the soil, rivers, lakes, oceans, and our food supply.

Fish and shellfish absorb mercury and store it in their fatty tissues. Mercury works its way up the food chain in a process called biomagnification as large fish eat smaller fish. The longer a fish lives, the more toxins like mercury it absorbs, and when you eat that fish you absorb it all. Almost all fish contain trace amounts of mercury, but the most contaminated fish are the predators at the top of the food chain, such as tuna, swordfish, shark, king mackerel, and tilefish. Mercury consumption from fish has been linked to brain and nervous system damage in unborn babies and young children, and has been found to cause cancer in rodents.[35]

FISHY FOOD

In 2003 the Environmental Working Group (EWG) released results of the extensive tests of cancer-causing PCB levels in farmed salmon consumed in the United States. EWG bought the salmon from local grocery stores and found 7 in 10 fish to be so contaminated with PCBs that they raised cancer-risk concerns, based on the health standards of the EPA.[36]

PCBs were banned in the U.S. in 1976 and have been linked to cancer and impaired fetal brain development. PCBs are stored in fatty tissue. Farmed salmon are fed fish meal that tends to be high in PCBs. As a result, farm-raised salmon has roughly 50 percent more fat than wild caught and averages 5 to 10 times more PCBs than wild-caught salmon.

Various species of wild fish have also been found to be contaminated with nanoparticles from the breakdown of plastics in our environment. These nanoparticles are able to cross the blood-brain barrier and cause brain damage and behavioral disorders in fish. Their effect on humans is not yet known.

WE ARE OVERFED BUT UNDERNOURISHED

We're stuffed, but we're starving. We're getting plenty of macronutrients (protein, fat, and carbs), but not nearly enough micronutrients like vitamins, minerals, enzymes, antioxidants, and the thousands of protective anti-cancer phytonutrients in plants, such as polyphenols, flavonoids, and carotenoids; allicin in garlic and onions; quercetin in apples; curcumin in turmeric; apigenin in celery; sulforaphane and indole-3-carbinol in broccoli; catechins in green tea; and ellagic acid in berries. These compounds are known to prevent cancers from forming, prevent tumors from growing, prevent cancer cells from spreading, and even directly cause cancer cell death. Fewer than 2 percent of Americans are getting the recommended minimum daily intake of potassium (4700mg).[37]

BURGER KINGS (AND QUEENS)

If you examine the life spans of the kings of Europe throughout history, you will see that many of them had short life spans. Rich people got rich people disease. Wealthy people got gout, heart disease, diabetes, and cancer because of their diets, which today would also be considered "whole foods" and "organic." Our wealthiest ancestors were also often obese. At one point in history, obesity was a status symbol, a sign of wealth, and obese women were considered the most beautiful because obesity implied a higher socioeconomic status and a life of leisure.

Kings and queens eat whatever they want, whenever they want. They can afford to eat three or more times per day, and they can eat expensive delicacies like meats and cheeses at every meal. Kings and queens can eat the finest, richest foods every day, foods rich in fat, sugar, salt, butter, cream, and oils. They have access to all the wine, beer, and spirits they desire. A king's diet is not a healthy diet. And it is no longer reserved for the wealthy. Today most Americans eat a diet high in animal products and sugar. Even worse, we're eating factory-farmed animal products and processed food loaded with man-made artificial additives, preservatives, flavors, and colors, as well as genetically modified food.

Historically, for the poor, meat was a luxury and typically only consumed on special occasions. Poor folks ate mostly plant foods like fruits, vegetables, legumes, and whole grains. This is still true today in undeveloped parts of the world. But in industrialized nations, thanks to large-scale factory farming and government subsidies that keep the prices of meat and sugar cheap, people can eat as much meat and sugar as they want. We are eating animal products and processed sugar at every meal and between meals. In the last century, processed sugar consumption has increased from about 4 pounds per person per year to roughly 100 pounds. That means the average person is eating about a pound of processed sugar every three days. We are eating about twice as much meat (6 times more chicken) and 25 times more sugar than our great-grandparents did in the early 1900s.[38]

If we keep eating the way we're eating, we're going to keep getting the diseases we're getting. If you eat a king's diet, you're going to get a king's diseases.

IS CANCER CONTAGIOUS?

According to the International Agency for Research on Cancer, 18 to 20 percent of cancers are linked to infections from cancer-causing viruses, such as hepatitis B and C, human immunodeficiency virus (HIV), some types of human papillomavirus (HPV), Epstein-Barr, and lesser known viruses like human T cell lymphotropic virus, Merkel cell polyomavirus, Kaposi sarcoma herpes virus, and bovine leukemia virus (BLV).[39]

Epstein-Barr virus, which has infected 95 percent of adults, has been found to cause Burkitt's lymphoma, Hodgkin's and non-Hodgkin's lymphoma, T cell lymphoma, nasopharyngeal cancer, and some cases of stomach cancer.[40]

Acute lymphoblastic leukemia, the most common form of childhood leukemia, has been linked to congenital cytomegalovirus (CMV), a form of herpes that can be passed from mother to child during childbirth. According to a study published in 2016, children born with congenital CMV are roughly four to six times more likely to develop ALL between two and six years old.[41] Fifty to eighty percent of American adults are infected with CMV by age 40, and one out of three pregnant women passes the virus to her unborn child.[42]

BLV is a cancer-causing virus found in cow's milk and meat. When milk supplies were tested in 2007, researchers discovered that 83 percent of small dairy farms and 100 percent of large dairy farms were found to be infected with bovine leukemia virus.[43] A human study found that 74 percent of subjects had antibodies indicating they had been previously exposed to BLV.[44] Pasteurization is thought to render BLV harmless in dairy products, but humans can also contract it from eating undercooked beef.[45]

In 2014, researchers identified BLV DNA in 44 percent of breast cancer tissue samples removed by surgery.[46] In 2015, they conducted another study to determine whether there was a link between BLV DNA in breast tissue and breast cancer, and concluded that the presence of BLV DNA in breast cancer tissue was strongly associated with diagnosed and histologically confirmed breast cancer. As many as 37 percent of breast cancer cases may be attributable to BLV exposure.[47]

Some viruses can't be avoided, but if you engage in risky behavior, such as unprotected sex or sharing needles with intravenous drugs, your odds of contracting multiple cancer-causing viruses are much higher. If your immune system is strong, your risk of developing cancer from viral infections is low, but viruses can lie dormant in your body for many years and then flare up if your immune system becomes weakened or suppressed for a prolonged period of time. This is why the factors in your life that you can control, like your diet, lifestyle, environment, and stress, are so important. A healthy body keeps infections in check.

CANCER RATES VARY GREATLY

The top cancers in Western nations are lung, colon, breast, and prostate cancer. In 1955, the death rate for pancreatic cancer, leukemia, and lymphomas was three to four times lower in Japan than in the United States, and the death rate for colon, prostate, breast, and ovarian cancers was five to ten times lower. This was at a time when animal products accounted for less than 5 percent of the Japanese diet.[48]

The Japan of 1955 was not an anomaly. Even today there are many parts of the world with much lower rates of cancer than are found in Western industrialized nations. Mexico has half the overall cancer rates of the United States. There are dozens of countries with a third of the overall cancer rates of the U.S.[49] In specific regions, and for specific cancers, it's even lower. The rate of colon cancer is over 60 times lower in native Africans than in African Americans.[50] The native Africans don't have a genetic advantage. They have a dietary advantage. They're not eating a Western diet, known to cause colon cancer.

To sum it up, we're sick. In the last 100 years, the incidence of chronic diseases such as cancer, heart disease, and diabetes has exploded in Western industrialized nations. It is clear that we have multiple factors working against us, including environmental pollution, a diet high in processed food and animal products, and a sedentary lifestyle. Scientists and researchers have identified the major causes of and contributors to chronic Western diseases, yet we are doing very little to prevent them. If you have a chronic disease like cancer or you are serious about prevention, the best thing you can do to promote health and healing in your body is to systematically identify and eliminate all of the cancer causers in your life and return to living as closely to nature as possible. True health care is self-care, taking care of yourself, but unfortunately, the medical and pharmaceutical industries have hijacked the words "health care" to put a rosy spin on what they do, which is most accurately described as sick care. In the following chapters, you'll see how sick the health-care industry has become.

DOCTOR'S ORDERS

I firmly believe that if the whole materia medica, as now used,
could be sunk to the bottom of the sea,
it would be better for mankind—and all the worse for the fishes.

— OLIVER WENDELL HOLMES

*P*RIMUM NON NOCERE. FIRST, DO NO HARM. This foundational principle of medical ethics dates back to Hippocrates, the father
of modern medicine. From the Hippocratic Corpus in *Epidemics*:
"The physician must . . . have two special objects in view with
regard to disease, namely, to do good or to do no harm." If the
methods involved in attempting to cure could produce more suffering than the disease itself, it's better to do nothing than to do
something that can potentially hurt a patient.

Most of us assume the best treatment options are the ones our
doctor recommends, but treating disease (not curing disease) is
a trillion-dollar-per-year global industry. Treating disease makes
doctors and drug companies a lot of money. The medical industry
needs a steady stream of sick people to stay in business. I'm not

implying that they want us to be sick or that they deliberately keep us sick, but the truth is that the medical industry benefits from our sickness. The sicker we all get, the more money they make.

Doctors are humans just like the rest of us, and sometimes humans are lazy, irresponsible, and negligent. I'm not demonizing doctors. There are many doctors who have had a positive impact on my life and to whom I owe a huge debt of gratitude. But let's be realistic. Earning a medical degree does not make you an ethical or moral person. There are good people and bad people in the world. Doctors are no exception. Some doctors care more about people, and some care more about money. Sometimes their priorities change over time. And sometimes it's hard to tell the difference.

Can you imagine being falsely diagnosed with cancer and then treated with multiple rounds of chemo? That is exactly what happened to the patients of Dr. Farid Fata in Michigan. Affectionately known as "Dr. Death," Fata was the perpetrator of one of the largest health-care frauds in American history. Over a six-year period, he falsely diagnosed or intentionally overtreated 553 people, fraudulently billed Medicare to the tune of $34 million dollars, laundered money, and engaged in a kickback scheme. Fata was busted in 2013, pleaded guilty, and was sentenced to 45 years in prison. And many of his patients/victims liked him and believed he was a good doctor. We have been conditioned to regard doctors as saintly, even superhuman. But they are not. They have the same flaws and problems as everyone else.

Being a doctor is a much harder job than most people realize. So hard that doctors have a higher rate of suicide than the general population. Male physicians have a 70 percent higher rate and female physicians have a 250 percent higher rate of suicide than everyone else.[1] Suicide is one of the leading causes of death for medical residents.[2] On a related note, more than 1 in 10 physicians develop drug and/or alcohol problems during their careers.[3] As scary as the implications of this are, let's not forget that sober doctors make mistakes too. But even if all doctors were saints and incapable of error, we would still have the same problem because for the most part, the problem is not doctors; it is our medical system, which is heavily influenced—some would say controlled—by the pharmaceutical industry.

DEATH BY MEDICINE

The third leading cause of death in the U.S. is a term most people have never heard of: iatrogenesis. That is death as a result of medical treatment. In 2000, a *JAMA* article reported that 225,000 Americans were dying each year from medical treatments.[4] Little has changed since then. In 2016, medical safety researchers at Johns Hopkins estimated that more than 250,000 deaths per year were due to medical errors.[5]

Here is an approximate break down of the iatrogenic deaths in the U.S. each year:

➤ Over 12,000 people die from unnecessary surgery.

➤ Over 7,000 people die from medication errors or negligence in hospitals.

➤ Over 20,000 people die from other hospital errors, like surgical errors.

➤ Over 90,000 people die from hospital-acquired infections.

➤ Over 127,000 people die from non-error prescription drug reactions.

Non-error prescription drug reactions are now the fourth leading cause of death in the United States. That's non-error. Every year over 127,000 people who are taking the correct doses of drugs prescribed to them by their doctors are dying from reactions to those drugs.[6,7]

Some experts believe that these numbers are inaccurately low because of unreliable "cause of death" reporting. Hospitals and doctors have a financial incentive (i.e., lawsuit avoidance) not to admit that they accidentally or unintentionally kill people, which is why they may decide to label a patient's cause of death as heart failure instead of heart failure from a drug reaction, or death from "cancer" instead of chemo toxicity.

One paper estimated that the number of medical deaths might be greater than 400,000 per year.[8] Another paper, entitled "Death by Medicine" and authored by Gary Null, Ph.D., Carolyn Dean, M.D., Martin Feldman, M.D., and colleagues, calculated the total number of iatrogenic deaths to be over three times higher than industry estimates, at 783,936 per year.[9,10] If their findings are correct, medical treatment is actually the number one killer of Americans. Even the seemingly harmless saline IV bags used in hospitals have been identified as contributors to kidney failure and death. Researchers estimate that 50,000 to 75,000 deaths could be prevented in the U.S. each year simply by replacing saline IV bags with balanced fluids such as lactated Ringer's solution or Plasma-Lyte A, which more closely mirror blood plasma and include electrolytes such as potassium and magnesium.[11] Your local hospital may be more dangerous than skid row, and the all too common scenario for patients who survive the gauntlet of medical treatment is that they find themselves trapped in a medical spin cycle of unnecessary tests, drugs, and procedures thanks to our epidemic of overdiagnosis and overtreatment.

DIAGNOSIS EPIDEMIC

Each year, tens of thousands of people, mostly women, undergo potentially harmful, unnecessary, and sometimes disfiguring treatments for precancerous conditions known as "incidentalomas." These are slow-growing, nonaggressive, indolent cancers or lesions that are unlikely to ever cause any harm. In 2014, Canadian researchers dropped a bombshell on the breast cancer industry via the *British Medical Journal (BMJ)*. Their 25-year study of nearly 90,000 women ages 45 to 59 found that mammograms made no difference in the breast cancer death rate when compared to physical breast exams.[12] For every woman saved by breast cancer screening, 10 women will be treated unnecessarily. According to a 2012 study published in *The New England Journal of Medicine*, mammograms have overdiagnosed 1.3 million women in the United States in the last 30 years.[13] It's estimated that for every breast cancer death prevented by a mammogram, there are one to three deaths caused by unnecessary treatments given to overdiagnosed women. This includes death from things like drug reactions or from the long-term effects of radiation therapy, which increases a women's risk for lung cancer and heart disease.

Since 1975, the number of new papillary thyroid cancer cases has nearly tripled, but the death rate has remained the same, at 0.5 per 100,000 people. The vast majority of these thyroid cancers were not life threatening, and thousands of people have been treated unnecessarily. Many have had their thyroids completely removed and now have no choice but to take hormone replacement drugs for the rest of their lives. In a 2014 *JAMA* paper, Louise Davies, M.D., found that the increase in thyroid cancer in women was nearly four times greater than in men and concluded, "There is an ongoing epidemic of thyroid cancer in the United States. The epidemiology of the increased incidence, however, suggests that it is not an epidemic of disease but rather an epidemic of diagnosis."[14]

Overdiagnosis and overtreatment for nonthreatening conditions liberally labeled as cancer have become such a serious issue that a panel of experts, including some of the top scientists in cancer research from the National Cancer Institute, published an article in *JAMA* taking the firm stance that increased screening has not improved the cancer death rate.[15] They also recommended redefining what medical conditions should even be called "cancer." Their opinion is that conditions such as ductal carcinoma in situ (DCIS), prostatic intraepithelial neoplasia, and lesions detected during breast, thyroid, lung, esophagus (Barrett's), and other cancer screenings should be reclassified as IDLE (indolent lesions of epithelial origin), removing all connection to cancer. In short, what many doctors are calling "cancer" today may, in the near future, be simply described as "a lesion that is not likely to spread." In response to the overdiagnosis problem, the American

Cancer Society updated its mammogram screening recommendations in 2018, pushing the starting age from 40 to 45, due to the high incidence of false positives for women under 45.

Another overdiagnosis revelation came from a 2013 study published in *JAMA*, which found that the lung cancer diagnosis rate was 11 percent higher with CT scans over X-rays, and that one in five lung tumors found on CT scans are indolent—growing so slowly that they are unlikely to cause a patient any problems at all. The study also reported that 320 patients have to get a CT screening to prevent one cancer death, and suggested that for every 10 lives saved by CT lung cancer screening, almost 14 people will have been diagnosed with a lung cancer that would never have caused any harm.[16] This indicates that as many as 2 of every 10 lung cancer patients are suffering financially, emotionally, and physically, and in some cases dying from side effects of unnecessary treatments. Lung cancer is the number one cancer killer, with a five-year survival rate of only about 17 percent, and many five-year survivors still have cancer. The small percentage of lung cancer patients who are permanently "cured" may only be so because they were misdiagnosed and treated for a disease that was not life threatening to begin with.

If you are diagnosed with cancer in the United States, your doctor can only prescribe a combination of surgery, drugs, and radiation. That's the "standard of care" in which every patient is essentially treated the same way. In most cases, your doctor is not allowed to prescribe a change in diet or lifestyle or any other natural or nontoxic therapy as a first-line therapy if you have been diagnosed with cancer. They can recommend dietary and lifestyle interventions and other therapies as "complementary" but often do not. And even though many doctors will acknowledge that the body is capable of healing itself, there are pervasive ignorance and arrogance in the medical community, which scoffs at natural healing methods, including evidence-based nutrition and lifestyle medicine.

The medical industry tends to view cancer in a linear fashion, like an unstoppable train. The assumption is that if you have cancer, your body is incapable of healing it. But there is actually a medical term for cancers that go away on their own. It's called spontaneous remission. In 1993, The Institute of Noetic Sciences published *Spontaneous Remission: An Annotated Bibliography*, documenting 3,500 medically reported spontaneous remissions from 800 medical journals in 20 different languages. After interviewing and studying many of these patients, Dr. Kelly Turner wrote a phenomenal book on the subject called *Radical Remission*. When cancer goes away on its own, the industry calls it spontaneous remission, but there's another word for it: *healing*. The body creates cancer and the body can heal it.

THE FEAR FACTORY

Many patients are told by their doctors that nothing they did contributed to their condition, that it was just "bad luck" or genetics. If you believe that you are powerless and there is nothing you can do to help yourself and promote health and healing in your body, then medical procedures and pharmaceutical drugs are your only hope.

Once cancer patients are convinced that oncology is their only hope, doctors often use fear to motivate them to take immediate action. They want to get you onto the conveyor belt as quickly as possible. And once you are strapped on, it is very difficult to get off. Fear is one of the strongest motivators there is, especially the fear of dying. When Micah and I met with the first oncologist, his message was clear. If I didn't do what he said, I was going to die. He was my only hope and nothing else would help me. I was terrified when I left the cancer clinic, and I began second-guessing my nutritional approach. Had I not already started to read and research on my own, I probably would have done what most cancer patients do: reluctantly show up for chemo out of fear.

COMMUNICATION BREAKDOWN

A 2012 study showed that 70 to 80 percent of terminal lung and colorectal cancer patients surveyed thought that the treatments they were receiving were likely to cure them, when in fact the patients were only given chemo as palliative care to "buy some time" or "improve their quality of life," with no intention of curing their cancer.[17]

When doctors were questioned about their failure to communicate the difference between curative and palliative care, a common excuse was "It's hard to tell patients that you can't cure their cancer." Doctors also have a financial incentive not to tell patients the whole truth. If oncologists told every terminal cancer patient that chemotherapy was not likely to cure them, and detailed how harmful and damaging the side effects would be, they would risk losing a lot of patients and a lot of income. Oncologists often use convoluted terminology, medical jargon, and positive-sounding words like "benefit," "successful," "effective," and "working" to describe cancer treatment, but what those words mean to a patient and to an oncologist are very different things.

It's common for patients to hear things like "Your type of cancer has shown to respond favorably to (insert drug therapy here)" or "This treatment has been shown to be effective and works well with your type of cancer." When a chemo drug is described as effective, beneficial, working, or successful, it usually only means the drug might shrink a tumor, or reduce the number of cancer cells in your body temporarily. If shrinkage happens, your cancer is "responding" to treatment. After treatment, it's not unusual for tumors to start growing again at a more aggressive pace. That's when the patient realizes that the "successful treatment" that shrank their tumor for a few months didn't produce the kind of success they were hoping for—curing their cancer.

To convolute further, the benefits of chemotherapy drugs are typically stated using relative risk percentages instead of absolute risk, or overall survival risk. This makes treatments appear more attractive. For example, let's say that after surgery a patient has a

6 percent risk of recurrence within five years, and the patient is told that the recommended chemo regimen has been shown to reduce her absolute or overall risk of recurrence from 6 percent to 3 percent. That patient might be inclined to pass on chemotherapy because her risk of recurrence after surgery is already low at only 6 percent.

But this same therapy that reduces absolute risk of recurrence from 6 percent to 3 percent can also be described as reducing relative risk of recurrence by 50 percent, which sounds huge. This is often how pharmaceutical sales reps sell new drugs to physicians, who in turn use the same statistics and language to sell drugs to patients. When a doctor tells a patient that a drug therapy can reduce her risk of recurrence by 50 percent, she will be far more inclined to say yes to treatment, not knowing that she is only reducing her absolute risk from 6 percent to 3 percent. But even if an oncologist does disclose the overall survival risk, most patients still have no idea what that means. Because it's all about context.

Your doctor tells you, "This combination of drugs is the most effective, and has been shown to increase overall survival in patients with your type of cancer." That sounds positive, but here's the terminology twist: "increasing overall survival" does not mean anyone actually survived. It may only mean that some patients lived a few weeks or a few months longer on that combo of drugs compared to another combo before dying. Furthermore, living an extra two months while being poisoned, sick, bedridden, and in and out of the hospital is not what most people would call living: more like living hell.

Even the term "remission" can be deceptive. Some oncologists use the term remission without distinguishing between partial remission and complete remission. Partial remission means the tumor shrunk partially. Complete remission means that cancer lesions, tumors, or cells are not detectable by scans or tests at a singular point in time, usually immediately after a round of treatments is complete. It's not uncommon for a cancer patient to achieve complete remission after being "successfully treated" with surgery, chemo, and radiation, only to have new tumors form soon thereafter because the underlying causes of cancer were not addressed.

In a recent study, researchers reported that complete remission rates were 76.5 percent for a subset of obese patients with acute myeloid leukemia. Remarkable, right? Not so fast. If you read a bit further, the authors disclose that the average survival of these patients was only 14 months.[18] Complete remission often only means that tumors are gone temporarily, not that cancer is cured. It takes years to determine whether a complete remission will become a permanent cure. Yet it is perfectly acceptable for an oncologist to tell an obese leukemia patient that chemotherapy treatment for AML achieves complete remission in 76 percent of cases. What patient wouldn't agree to a treatment with a 76 percent remission rate? To the patient, a 76 percent remission rate means a 76 percent *cure* rate. But the oncologist knows the cancer is likely to come back after treatment and that the patient will probably die in one to two years. And they may not disclose that to the patient because "It's hard to tell patients you can't cure their cancer."

DOES TREATMENT REALLY EXTEND LIFE?

Over many decades, the cancer industry has developed a unique way of rebranding its failures as successes. To you and me, a successful treatment means being cured of cancer with no recurrence. Complete long-term restoration of health is success. Sickness and death are failure. In the cancer industry, success is measured in a variety of ways that are all designed to reflect positively on the industry. Tiny improvements are heralded as huge successes. One of these is "life extension." If you live a few months longer than your prognosis, which is a guess based on averages, then your treatment "worked" and was a "success," even if you die. Many studies demonstrating life extension of a drug therapy do not have control groups of patients who did no therapy at all.

In 1992, Dr. Ulrich Abel at the University of Heidelberg, Germany, published a comprehensive 92-page analysis of every available clinical trial and publication examining the value of chemotherapy in treating advanced epithelial cancers, also known as carcinomas. These are responsible for more than 80 percent of cancer deaths worldwide, including nearly all malignant tumors of the head, neck, lung, breast, bladder, colon, rectum, pancreas, ovary, cervix, and liver. His research also included surveying hundreds of oncologists around the world. A condensed version of his analysis, which included 140 citations, was published as an article in *Biomedicine & Pharmacotherapy*. Here's an excerpt from Abel's summary:

> Apart from lung cancer, in particular small cell lung cancer, there is no direct evidence that chemotherapy prolongs survival in patients with advanced carcinoma. . . . Many oncologists take it for granted that response to therapy prolongs survival, an opinion which is based on fallacy and which is not supported by clinical studies. . . . With few exceptions, there is no good scientific basis for the application of chemotherapy in symptom-free patients with advanced epithelial malignancy.[19]

Abel's exhaustive and virtually irrefutable research made little to no measurable impact on the cancer industry's standard of care in the years that followed.

In the United States, cancer is the second leading cause of death behind heart disease, and is predicted to be number one soon as it is now the leading cause of death in 22 states. Despite the many innovations in drugs and treatments in the last half century, the cancer industry has not improved the death rate for most cancers, especially epithelial solid tumor cancers. Lung cancer is the number one cancer killer in the U.S., claiming roughly 150,000 people each year. Today, decades after Abel's analysis, standard chemo treatment for non–small cell lung cancer, which is 85 to 90 percent of lung cancers, costs over $40,000 and may only give a patient an extra two months of life. More than half of people with lung cancer die within one year of being diagnosed.[20,21] The average survival of untreated lung cancer patients is seven months.[22]

Defenders of oncology are quick to dismiss older studies such as Abel's as irrelevant due to the development of new drugs and improvements in treatment methods, while conveniently neglecting to mention that some of the most popular chemotherapy drugs used today are between 20 and 60 years old. Here's a list of ten of the most commonly prescribed chemo drugs and when they were developed:

- ➤ Methotrexate —1950s
- ➤ Fluorouracil (5-FU)—1957
- ➤ Cyclophosphamide (Cytoxan, Neosar)—1959
- ➤ Doxorubicin (Adriamycin)—1960s
- ➤ Cisplatin (Platinol)—1978
- ➤ Gemcitabine (Gemzar)—1980s
- ➤ Etoposide (Eposin, Etopophos, VePesid, VP-16)—1983
- ➤ Chlorambucil (Leukeran)—pre-1984
- ➤ Docetaxel (Taxotere, Docecad)—1992
- ➤ Paclitaxel (Taxol, Abraxane)—1992

In 2013 a study reported that the proportion of patients in the Netherlands with metastatic gastric cancer increased from 24 percent in 1990 to 44 percent in 2011. The use of palliative chemotherapy to treat it increased from 5 percent to 36 percent during this time period, with "a strong increase" after 2006.[23] In this time period, the metastatic gastric cancer rate doubled and the use of chemo for it increased sevenfold, but the average overall survival only increased from 15 weeks in 1990 to 17 weeks in 2011. Twenty-one years of advancements in cancer treatment might get you an extra two weeks of life if you have metastatic gastric cancer. Yet the authors of the study still found a way to put a positive spin on the results by stating that "overall survival remained stable."

A study published in *JAMA* in 2015 reported that giving chemotherapy to end-stage cancer patients with fewer than six months to live did not improve their survival or their quality of life. The sickest patients had no benefit and those who weren't as sick suffered more. The patients who opted out of chemo lived just as long and had better quality of life than those who took the chemo.[24]

Unfortunately, Hippocrates's principle "First, do no harm" has been abandoned by the cancer industry, and treatments are often prescribed despite the certainty of severe physical damage and life-threatening risk to the patient. Most chemotherapy drugs have the potential to cause substantial harm and are often given to the point of overwhelming toxicity, with an all too common end result of death, especially for metastatic solid tumor cancers. So if studies and statistics have shown the same underwhelming results time and time again, why in the world would conventional medicine continue prescribing treatments that don't permanently cure most cancers?

MAKING
A KILLING

Good health makes a lot of sense,
but it doesn't make a lot of dollars.

— DR. ANDREW SAUL

IN 1897 SCIENTISTS AT BAYER began experimenting with acetyl-salicylic acid, an extract from the bark of the willow tree, known for centuries to be a pain reliever. They discovered a new way to synthesize it, patented the formula, and two years later began selling it as aspirin. And the rest is history. Aspirin quickly became the biggest drug in the world and ushered in a new era of pharmaceutical medicine, which is now a trillion-dollar industry. Pharmaceutical companies make money by creating unique drugs that can be patented and sold at high profits for many years with no competition. Over the past century, the pharmaceutical industry has infiltrated every aspect of medicine and exerts enormous influence over the health-care industry, or what is known as the medical-industrial complex.

"The medical profession is being bought by the pharmaceutical industry, not only in terms of the practice of medicine, but also in terms of teaching and research. The academic institutions of this country are allowing themselves to be the paid agents of the pharmaceutical industry. I think it's disgraceful."

— DR. ARNOLD S. RELMAN,
former editor-in-chief of *The New England Journal of Medicine,* who coined the term "medical-industrial complex"

In the United States, medical doctors get their educations and earn their degrees at institutions funded by drug companies. Doctors are certified by the American Medical Association (AMA), which receives funding from the drug companies. Doctors prescribe drugs approved by the Food and Drug Administration (FDA), which receives roughly $100 million per year in "user fees" from drug companies for new drug applications. The pharmaceutical industry has over 1,200 registered lobbyists in Washington, D.C., and spent $900 million lobbying on legislation and $90 million in campaign contributions to politicians from 1998 to 2005 alone.[1] In 2003 the Bush administration passed Medicare Part D, which prohibits the federal government from negotiating prices with the pharmaceutical industry. This allows the drug companies to charge Medicare whatever prices they want. In addition, Medicare and private health insurers waste nearly $3 billion every year throwing away unused cancer medicines because many drug makers distribute the drugs in one-size-fits-all vials with a dose that is too large for most patients; the unused drugs get tossed in the trash.[2]

There are only three countries in the world that allow drug companies to advertise to consumers: the United States, New Zealand, and to a lesser extent, Canada. In the States, drug ads are everywhere: on TV, on billboards, in magazines, and online. How did this happen? Lobbying. Decades of lobbying have led to government legislation that funnels American tax dollars directly to the drug companies. Pharmaceutical companies create their own philanthropies, fund research to create and patent drugs with tax-exempt dollars, sell themselves the patents to the drugs, and then sell those drugs to the public.

We the taxpayers fund the research; then the drug companies make billions in profit selling the drugs back to us. The U.S. government spent $484 million developing the cancer drug Taxol and then licensed it to Bristol-Myers Squibb, which has made over $9 billion on the drug and only paid $35 million in royalties to the National Institutes of Health.[3]

The pharmaceutical industry has spent billions of dollars to convince Americans that patented drugs are the answer to all of our ailments, but in most cases of chronic disease drugs don't cure us. They only alleviate some of the symptoms of disease, enabling us to continue the behaviors that are making us sick. Drugs make our sickness tolerable so we are able to function while unwell, in a state of "vertical illness." And they create long-term dependence. They've made us addicts.

MEDICATION NATION

We the people are heavily medicated. Half of Americans are taking one prescription drug monthly, 21 percent are taking three or more, and 10 percent of us are taking more than five prescription drugs per month. And Americans now pay twice as much for prescription drugs on average than the citizens of any other developed country.[4]

Many prescription drugs have side effects that can cause new problems with long-term use, creating a vicious cycle in which patients are taking drugs for the side effects of drugs, and then more drugs for the side effects of those drugs. Some prescription drugs are highly addictive, while others help just enough to perpetuate continual use. It seems that the strategy of the drug marketers—and it has been remarkably successful—is to convince Americans that there are only two kinds of people: those with medical conditions that require drug treatment and those who don't know it yet.[5]

In the United States alone, the number of prescriptions written for painkillers nearly tripled from 1990 to 2010. There were 209.5 million painkiller prescriptions written in 2010 alone, enough to medicate every single American all day and night for an entire month. As a result, the number of unintentional overdoses has quadrupled.[6] Prescription drug reactions are the seventh leading cause of death in the United States, killing over 100,000 people every year. Opioid painkillers like methadone, oxycodone, and hydrocodone are killing more people than cocaine and heroin combined. As bad as the opioid epidemic is, surprisingly only about 15 percent of prescription drug deaths are from painkillers. Roughly 85,000 deaths per year are caused by all the other drugs we are taking. Those prescription meds with a "low risk of side effects" in your medicine cabinet may not be so low risk after all. Fun fact: Bayer used to sell heroin as cough medicine.

For the better part of the last century, the pharmaceutical industry has enjoyed a monopoly on medicine and the public trust. But in the last two decades, the rise of the internet and widespread access to information have led to a collective consciousness of the pitfalls and perils of conventional medicine and to a resurgence in the interest in and use of nutrition and natural, nontoxic therapies for healing and preventing disease. In response to the natural health movement, pharmaceutical-based medicine rebranded itself as "science-based medicine" and "evidence-based medicine," using the word "science" to imply truth and the word "evidence" to imply proof. Like all manufactured goods, it goes without saying that there is science involved. Of course drugs are science-based, and so are Pop-Tarts. When it comes to evidence-based medicine, however, in some cases, the more closely you look the less you find.

Pharmaceutical medicine is most accurately described as patent-based, profit-based medicine because drug companies are only interested in evidence that can lead to patented, highly profitable pharmaceutical drugs. Over 100,000 nutritional science studies are published each year and for the most part ignored by the medical and pharmaceutical industry, despite the fact that these studies continue to contribute to the mountain of evidence that many of the leading causes of premature death from chronic disease (such as heart disease, diabetes, cancer) can be prevented and reversed through simple, inexpensive diet and lifestyle changes. The pharmaceutical and medical industries ignore this information because it isn't profitable. They can't make billions of dollars prescribing diet and lifestyle interventions like nutrition, exercise, and stress reduction. So they only focus on evidence that can produce patentable drugs. The inherent implication of evidence-based medicine is that it must have strong scientific evidence behind it. But that's not always the case. A large-scale meta-analysis of published and unpublished antidepressant drug trials found that placebos worked as well as the drugs 82 percent of the time![7] In addition, 57 percent of the drug trials failed to show any benefit, but most of those trials were not published.

In March 2012 C. Glenn Begley, a former head of global cancer research at pharmaceutical giant Amgen, reported that during the 10 years he spent at Amgen, he and his team of 100 scientists discovered that 47 of 53 "landmark" cancer studies could not be replicated, in some cases after 50 attempts.[8] Amgen's intention was to verify the reliability of the 53 studies before spending millions of dollars to develop new drugs based on them. Here's what Begley had to say about their findings:

> It was shocking. . . . These are the studies the pharmaceutical industry relies on to identify new targets for drug development. But if you're going to place a $1 million, or $2 million, or $5 million bet on an observation, you need to be sure it's true. As we tried to reproduce these papers we became convinced you can't take anything at face value.[9]

Our favorite heroin cough syrup makers, Bayer AG, published a similar report entitled "Believe It or Not," in which they revealed that less than a fourth of 47 cancer projects undertaken in 2011 reproduced the findings of previously published research, despite the efforts of three or four scientists working full-time for up to a year. Those projects were dropped.[10]

The failed replication projects at Amgen and Bayer clearly indicate that many of the "landmark" scientific studies that have significantly influenced cancer drug development and treatment were either flukes or fakes. The incentives to publish nonreplicable drug studies can be traced to both the pharmaceutical companies and the researchers themselves. With increasing competition for academic jobs and research funding, getting published in a scientific journal can be a significant career booster, resulting in job security, bonuses, research grants, and job offers. Thus if a researcher conducted the same experiment ten times and only got a positive result once, he could ignore the nine times it didn't work and publish findings on the one time it did—the fluke. And no one is the wiser until an attempt is made to replicate the study. The fakes, in contrast, occur when researchers falsify or manipulate data to support their hypothesis or achieve a desired outcome, such as proving that a drug works.

In 2006 alone nearly one-third of 1,534 cancer research papers published in major journals disclosed that the study was either funded by the pharmaceutical industry or conducted by an industry employee. These studies were more likely to have positive findings, indicating that researchers were biased toward their industry connections.[11] Between 2001 and 2010, the number of published journal articles increased by about 44 percent but the number of scientific papers that had to be retracted increased by over 1,000 percent. A review of over 2,000 retracted papers found that only 21 percent were due to errors and 67 percent of retractions were due to fraud or suspected fraud and plagiarism.[12] Consider the opinions of the editors in chief of two the most prestigious and well-respected medical journals in the world.

> The case against science is straightforward: much of the scientific literature, perhaps half, may simply be untrue. Afflicted by studies with small sample sizes, tiny effects, invalid exploratory analyses, and flagrant conflicts

of interest, together with an obsession for pursuing fashionable trends of dubious importance, science has taken a turn towards darkness.[13]

— DR. RICHARD HORTON,
editor-in-chief of *The Lancet*

It is simply no longer possible to believe much of the clinical research that is published, or to rely on the judgment of trusted physicians or authoritative medical guidelines. I take no pleasure in this conclusion, which I reached slowly and reluctantly over my two decades as an editor of *The New England Journal of Medicine.*"[14]

— DR. MARCIA ANGELL

In November 2013 it was reported that breast cancer patients taking paclitaxel, a 20-year-old generic drug, actually lived one to three months longer than patients taking "promising new drugs" Abraxane and Ixempra, which cost $4,000 to $5,000 per dose and had nearly $500 million in combined sales in 2012. The cheaper 20-year-old drug worked better. In this case, the word "better" is relative because the patients still died. The report also noted that patients taking any of those three drugs combined with Avastin typically had their cancer return or progress within seven to nine months.[15,16]

Inaccurate and incomplete scientific research leads to the development of drugs that don't work well, or at all. A 2017 study published in the *British Medical Journal* found that over half of the new cancer drugs approved in Europe between 2009 and 2013 showed no benefit. These expensive new drugs did not improve survival or even quality of life.[17,18] In some cases, hyped-up, evidence-less drugs rushed to market can cause serious damage and death.

One of the most egregious examples of the harm caused by "evidence-based" medicine used without actual evidence is Avastin. One of the world's top-selling cancer drugs at the time, Avastin was approved for use on metastatic breast cancer in 2008 under the FDA's accelerated approval program, which allows a drug to be fast-tracked even with insufficient data. After Avastin's approval, drug maker Genentech completed two clinical trials, only to find that the results could not back up their claims. In November 2011, the FDA revoked Avastin's approval for treatment of breast cancer after concluding that the drug was dangerous and didn't work. FDA commissioner Margaret Hamburg issued the following statement:

> After reviewing the available studies, it is clear that women who take Avastin for metastatic breast cancer risk potentially life-threatening side effects without proof that the use of Avastin will provide a benefit, in terms of delay in tumor growth, that would justify those risks. Nor is there evidence that use of Avastin will either help them live longer or improve their quality of life.[19]

For two and a half years, tens of thousands of women were pre-scribed Avastin for breast cancer and many of them suffered from its life-threatening effects, including severe high blood pressure, perforations in their stomach and intestines, internal bleeding, and hemorrhaging, as well as heart attacks, heart failure, and death.

In November 2014, the FDA approved Avastin for use in platinum-resistant recurrent ovarian cancer because Avastin was shown to reduce the risk of the disease worsening or death by 62 percent when used along with 60-year-old chemo drug paclitaxel, when compared to chemotherapy alone. According to Sandra Horning, M.D., head of Global Product Development for Genentech, "Avastin plus chemotherapy is the first new treatment option for women with this difficult-to-treat type of ovarian cancer in more than 15 years." An impressive claim, but the patients taking Avastin only lived about three and a half months longer on average.

Genentech brought in over $48 billion in net sales revenue between 2006 and 2014, largely from selling Avastin. The drug is still on the market today, approved for use for several other cancers and typically given to terminal cancer patients, hoping it might buy them a bit more time, at a cost of over $50,000 per year.

A recent study found that patients who took Avastin combined with chemotherapy had a 50 percent increased risk of dying from its complications versus those who received standard chemotherapy. Patients given Avastin along with platinum- or taxane-based chemotherapy agents, such as carboplatin or paclitaxel, had over triple the risk of dying.[20,21]

In 2016, Genentech and OSI Pharmaceuticals were ordered to pay a $67 million fine for giving promotional materials to oncologists that included misleading and overstated survival data about the effectiveness of Tarceva to treat non–small cell lung cancer. Oncologists were persuaded to prescribe Tarceva as a first-line therapy and were not informed that there was little evidence to show that the drug had any benefit unless the patient had never smoked or had a mutation in their epidermal growth factor receptor, which is a protein involved in the spread of cancer cells.[22,23]

THE 2 PERCENT STUDY

In 2004, my first year of cancer, a groundbreaking study was published in the *Journal of Clinical Oncology* examining the five-year survival rates of cancer patients in the U.S. and Australia. The study included over 154,000 Americans and 72,000 Australian adults with 22 types of cancer who were treated with chemotherapy.[24] The study's conclusion:

> The overall contribution of curative and adjuvant cytotoxic chemotherapy to 5-year survival in adults was estimated to be 2.3% in Australia and 2.1% in the USA. . . . As the 5-year relative survival rate in Australia is now over 60%, it is clear that cytotoxic chemotherapy only makes a minor contribution to cancer survival. To justify the continued funding and availability of drugs used in cytotoxic chemotherapy, a rigorous evaluation of the cost-effectiveness and impact on quality of life is urgently required.

In this study, only 3,306 of 154,971 American cancer patients had five-year survival that could be credited to chemotherapy. The study did not distinguish between the survivors who were NED (no evidence of disease) or AWD (alive with disease). The only thing we know is that 3,306 patients were still alive at the five-year mark. Patients in hospice and on life support are considered successfully treated five-year survivors as long as their hearts are beating at the five-year mark. It is likely that some of these five-year survivors still had cancer or had a recurrence in subsequent years and eventually died.

In fairness, averaging the five-year survival rates of 22 different cancers and claiming that "chemo only works 2 percent of the time" is misleading. This is not unlike when my first oncologist told me I had a 60 percent chance of living five years, which was the average survival of all cancer patients lumped together. According to this study, chemotherapy would have only contributed about 1 percent to my five-year survival for colon cancer, worse than the 2.1 percent average. To its credit, chemotherapy was found to increase five-year survival of testicular cancer by 40.3 percent and Hodgkin's disease by 37.7 percent. Chemotherapy also contributes to better five-year survival rates for childhood acute myeloid leukemia (85 percent), and rare cancers like Burkitt's lymphoma, which has a cure rate of over 90 percent. Those cancers were not included in this study.

A major factor impacting the conclusion of the 2 percent study was that the five-year survival benefit for many cancers after chemo treatment was zero. No survivors. The cancers for which chemo reportedly made no difference toward five-year survival were melanoma, multiple myeloma, and soft-tissue sarcoma, as well as pancreatic, uterine, prostate, bladder, and kidney cancers.

SIDE EFFECTS MAY INCLUDE . . .

Side effects of prescription drugs can sometimes be worse than the disease the drug is designed to treat and can increase your risk of cancer, and many other debilitating and life-threatening diseases, and death. All prescription drugs abnormally alter metabolic functions in your body and many cause additional health problems with extended use. For example, according to the disclaimer in a commercial for the arthritis drug Xeljanz, "Serious, sometimes fatal infections and cancers have happened in patients taking Xeljanz." The drug companies are telling us that their drugs can cause life-threatening infections and cancer, and we're taking them anyway.

Oral contraceptives (birth control pills) are classified as a Group 1 carcinogen, a special designation reserved for known cancer causers like cigarette smoking. In October 2006, the Mayo Clinic published a peer-reviewed meta-analysis that showed a 44 to 52 percent increased risk of premenopausal breast cancer in women who used oral contraceptives before their first full-term pregnancy. Women who used oral contraceptives for four or more years before their first full-term pregnancy had the highest risk.[25]

Sometimes pharmaceutical companies neglect to inform consumers of the potentially life-threatening side effects of their drugs and get in big trouble for it. In April 2014 a U.S. jury ordered Takeda Pharmaceutical Company Ltd and Eli Lilly and Company to pay a total of $9 billion in punitive damages for concealing the fact that their diabetes drug Actos increased cancer risk.

CANCER DRUGS CAN CAUSE CANCER

Many chemotherapy drugs are carcinogenic, which means they can cause new cancers in the body. Other chemo drugs, while not directly cancer causing, can severely damage your immune system, which can give existing cancers the opportunity to spread rapidly. Some of the chemotherapy drugs identified as carcinogenic by the U.S. National Toxicology Program are Adriamycin, chlorambucil, cisplatin, Cytoxan, dacarbazine, Leukeran, Mustargen, Myleran, nitrosourea agents (CCNU, BiCNU, Streptozotocin, STZ, Zanosar), melphalan, tamoxifen, and thiotepa.

Chemotherapy can also backfire and boost cancer growth. When healthy cells are damaged by chemotherapy, they can secrete a protein called WNT16B. This protein can feed existing tumors, helping them grow and making them resistant to further treatment, which is why approximately 90 percent of patients with solid metastatic cancers, including breast, prostate, lung, and colon cancer, develop resistance to chemotherapy.[26] Research published in 2017 found that when cancer cells are injured or killed by chemotherapy, targeted therapies, and radiotherapy, they trigger an inflammatory "cytokine storm" in the tumor microenvironment that sets the stage to promote new tumor growth.[27] Researchers in Israel had a similar finding. When they dripped the blood of patients treated with chemotherapy on cancer cells in the lab, it made those cancer cells more aggressive.[28] Despite these recent revelations, this is really not new information. Doctors and researchers have known that chemotherapy causes more aggressive cancers to spread throughout the body since chemotherapy was first introduced. One example is the cancer drug tamoxifen, which has been reported to reduce a woman's risk of a secondary estrogen receptor-positive breast cancer by 60 percent. But if the cancer returns, it is four times more likely to be a more aggressive, estrogen receptor-negative breast cancer.[29] Tamoxifen also increases a woman's risk for uterine cancer and potentially fatal blood clots.[30]

COLLATERAL DAMAGE

Chemotherapy drugs can cause damage throughout your body all the way down to your DNA. Many chemotherapy drugs carry an FDA "black box" warning because they can cause life-threatening side effects and death. Nurses who administer chemo drugs are required to wear protective gear to make sure they don't get these dangerous chemicals on their skin while they inject them into a patient's veins. If any chemo drugs spill on the floor, medical staff have to use a special kit to clean up the spill, which is at that point considered hazardous waste.

Most folks know that chemotherapy drugs can cause hair loss, but unfortunately for some cancer patients who took Taxotere (docetaxel), the drug caused permanent baldness. According to one lawsuit, drug maker Sanofi-Aventis allegedly knew that permanent hair loss was a potential side effect in 2005 but failed to disclose this to patients and doctors in the United States until 2016.[31]

One significant area of damage that chemo patients often suffer from is brain damage, which is known as "chemo brain" and marked by an inability to think clearly, organize thoughts, and concentrate. Chemo brain has been reported to affect as many as 70 percent of cancer patients, and severe symptoms include memory loss, mental and emotional instability, and even dementia. For years the industry claimed there was no such thing as chemo brain, until recent studies validated patients' claims.

Platinum-based chemo drugs like cisplatin and carboplatin are nephrotoxic, causing kidney damage, or ototoxic, causing temporary or permanent hearing loss. Drugs such as doxorubicin are cardiotoxic and can cause heart damage. Drugs like bleomycin and busulfan can cause pulmonary fibrosis, which is lung damage. Other chemo drugs such as methotrexate and 5-fluorouracil (5-FU) cause myelosuppression, which is bone marrow damage that decimates your immune system and in severe cases may require a bone marrow transplant.

Drugs in the vinca alkaloid family like vincristine and vinblastin can cause peripheral neuropathy, or nerve damage in your hands and feet, causing the loss of feeling and function. This can cripple you for life, and as a result some cancer patients are unable to feed, clothe, or bathe themselves.

Chemo drugs such as cyclophosphamide can cause hemorrhagic cystitis, resulting in bladder damage and permanent loss of bladder control. Chemo drugs can also induce early menopause in women and result in a significant loss in bone density in premenopausal women, increasing the risk of fractures. In severe cases, chemo drugs can cause potentially fatal blood clots or destroy your blood, requiring a blood transfusion. Chemo can also make both men and women sterile.

In early 2013, the FDA and Health Canada both issued warnings that in rare cases Avastin was linked to a life-threatening flesh-eating bacterial infection called necrotizing fasciitis.

WHAT ABOUT IMMUNOTHERAPY?

In recent years, immunotherapy drugs, which attempt to harness a patient's immune system to seek and destroy cancer cells, have been hailed as "a new hope," "a game changer," and "the biggest breakthrough since chemotherapy." Your immune system is vitally important in keeping you well and cancer free, and improving the immune system's ability to eliminate cancer is a step in the right direction for cancer therapy.

Immunotherapy is currently the hottest trend in the cancer treatment world, and as I write this, there are roughly 800 clinical trials under way using immunotherapy drugs, but the initial results do not justify the hype. Immunotherapy drugs only show a response rate in about 20 percent of patients for some cancers and have no effect on others. It's currently estimated that only 8 percent of cancer patients will get any benefit in terms of tumor shrinkage or delayed cancer progression from immunotherapy drugs.[32] And the risks with immunotherapy drugs can be just as severe and life threatening as chemo drugs. Patients in trials have died from reactions to immunotherapy drugs. Beyond that, the cost of these drugs is astronomical.

One example is a headline-making trial that reported that combining Yervoy and Opdivo to treat patients with melanoma increased median progression-free survival by 11.5 months, which was much better than either drug alone, but cost nearly $300,000 per patient. Coincidentally, only 11.5 percent of patients had complete remission during the trial. Sixty-five percent of the patients in the trial had to stop the therapy because of drug toxicity, disease progression, or death.[33]

Another trial on Opdivo for lung cancer reported that patients got an extra three months of life at a cost of $100,000. Based on that finding, Bristol-Meyers Squibb actually trademarked the slogan "A chance to live longer" for use in their Opdivo commercials, which also discloses that "Opdivo can cause your immune system to attack normal organs and tissues in any area of your body and can affect the way they work. These problems can sometimes become serious or life threatening and can lead to death." Another immunotherapy drug, Keytruda, is estimated to cost as much $1 million dollars per year, per patient, depending on the dose amount.[34] Merck and Bristol-Myers Squibb sold almost $9 billion worth of immunotherapy drugs between 2015 and 2017.[35]

RADIATION EXPLOSION

Radiation exposure in the U.S. population from diagnostic imaging has increased sixfold in the last 30 years, primarily due to the rapid increase in CT scans from 1 million per year to about 80 million per year. Ionizing radiation from CT scans is powerful enough to damage DNA, which can lead to cancer. But would you believe that one-third of the patients getting a CT scan didn't even know the test exposed their body to radiation? In a 2012 study, researchers found that 85 percent of patients underestimated the amount of radiation delivered by a CT scan and one-third of patients didn't know CT scans produced radiation at all.[36] On a personal level, I had no idea how much radiation was used in CT scans until I researched on my own. One CT of the abdomen and pelvis exposes you to as much radiation as 100 chest X-rays. A PET/CT combo is the equivalent of 250 chest X-rays.[37]

Radiation treatments are one of the top five causes of secondary cancers for cancer survivors. The most common radiation-related cancers are lung, breast, thyroid, stomach, and leukemia. Eight percent of secondary cancers are related to radiation therapy. The percentage is a bit higher for prostate cancer (11 percent), cervical cancer (18 percent), and testicular cancer (25 percent).

The radiation from a CT scan is considered to be twice as carcinogenic as the gamma rays from the atomic bombs dropped on Hiroshima and Nagasaki.[38] After only one CT scan, your risk of radiation-related cancer remains elevated throughout the rest of your life and your risk increases with every scan. It's estimated that diagnostic radiation causes 1 to 3 percent of all cancers and that the number of radiation-related cancers will triple in the coming years if diagnostic radiation use continues at current levels. A recent National Cancer Institute study estimates there will be about 29,000 future cancers as a result of scans done in 2007 alone.[39]

From 1995 to 2008, the use of CT scans on children at general hospitals increased by a factor of five. In children's hospitals, CT scan use increased by a factor of 13, from nearly 15,000 in 1995 to 200,000 in 2008.[40] Children are especially vulnerable to radiation damage. A 2012 study reported that a childhood CT scan (or scans) resulting in a cumulative exposure of 50 to 60 mGy (milligrays) of radiation before age 15 can nearly triple their risk of developing brain cancer and leukemia in the future.[41] The cancer risk from CT scans decreases significantly after age 25. Good evidence suggests that 20 to 50 percent of childhood CT scans could be replaced with another type of imaging or not done at all.

CT SCANS: RESULTS MAY VARY

In 2011 a team of researchers at Memorial Sloan Kettering Cancer Center took 30 patients with stage III or IV lung cancer and a minimum tumor size of 1 centimeter and gave them two CT scans 15 minutes apart. Three expert radiologists were on hand to read the scans and measure the tumors but were not told that the same patients were being scanned twice.

Nearly two-thirds of the patients had a measurable difference in tumor size of a millimeter or more, and a third of them had a difference of two millimeters. Some of the tumors shrunk by as much as 23 percent and some grew by as much as 31 percent.[42] Again, this was after only 15 minutes. So did the CT scan cause the cancers to shrink, or grow, or both?

None of the above. What this study demonstrated is that CT scans can be unreliable when measuring cancer progression. Measuring the diameter of a tumor perfectly in the center in scan #1, then measuring it slightly off center in scan #2, or vice versa, can lead to a discrepancy in size between the two scans. And a small discrepancy in a CT scan can have massive consequences.

For example, if a CT scan indicated that your tumor grew by 31 percent, you would assume that treatment is not working. In which case, your doctor might be prompted to recommend more aggressive treatment, which may be completely unnecessary and harmful. In reality, a scan showing up to a 30 percent change in tumor size may not mean anything at all. Even if your tumor did grow by 30 percent—although that sounds huge—this may only represent a change of a few millimeters. A 1 centimeter tumor that grew by 30 percent is still only 1.3 centimeters, which is tiny, and in many parts of the body would not be considered life threatening.

LITTLE-KNOWN RISKS OF RADIOTHERAPY

When radiotherapy shrinks a breast cancer tumor by 50 percent, everyone assumes that's a good thing, but researchers at UCLA discovered that the radiation often kills benign cells. It also makes the surviving breast cancer stem cells resistant to further treatment and up to 30 times more likely to form new tumors than the non-irradiated breast cancer cells.[43]

Another study found that ionizing radiation reprogrammed less-malignant breast cancer cells into breast cancer stem cells, creating treatment-resistant "super cells." Radiotherapy can not only make existing breast cancer stem cells stronger and more aggressive, but it can also create new breast cancer stem cells. Radiotherapy has also been found to increase cancer stem cells in the prostate, resulting in cancer recurrence and worsened prognosis.[44] Another commonly undisclosed side effect of chest radiotherapy, especially when treating breast cancer, is that it can cause significant damage to the heart and arteries, leading to heart disease.[45]

In 2004 a large randomized trial (CALGB 9343) found that women 70 and older with estrogen-positive and/or progesterone-positive stage I breast cancer had no increase in overall survival after radiation treatments. Five years after this study was published, nearly two-thirds of breast cancer patients over 70 were still being unnecessarily treated with radiation therapy.[46] According to study author Dr. Rachel Blitzblau, "We should consider omitting radiation for these women, because the small observed benefits might not be worth the side effects and costs."

WHAT ABOUT DENTAL X-RAYS?

All ionizing radiation is harmful, and small doses add up over time. Ionizing radiation from dental X-rays increases your risk for meningioma, the most common type of brain tumor. In a 2012 study of 1,433 cases, researchers reported that those who reported ever having a bitewing X-ray at any age had twice the risk of developing a brain tumor. Those who had a panoramic (panorex) full mouth X-ray before age 10 had nearly five times the risk.[47] In addition, there have been several studies linking dental X-rays to an increased risk of thyroid cancer. If you need to have a dental X-ray, make sure they use a neck shield. Also avoid the 3-D cone-beam CT, which uses about six times more radiation than traditional dental X-rays. The American Dental Association has acknowledged that routine dental X-rays are unnecessary, and that there is no need for dental X-rays on patients who are not having any pain or teeth problems.[48] In 2006, the *Journal of the American Dental Association* stated that "dentists should not prescribe routine X-rays at preset intervals for all patients." Yet many still do.

The conventional medical model is an approach that tends to treat symptoms of disease with drugs, surgery, radiation, or other procedures, rather than the causes of disease. These limited procedures are largely a one-size-fits-all approach to treatment, and doctors today have become highly specialized, treating only individual body parts rather than the whole body. Medical doctors do not have the freedom to practice medicine. Instead they have a strict set of guidelines they must follow. If they deviate from these guidelines, they risk losing their license to practice medicine and their livelihood.

The pharmaceutical industry is pulling the strings of the health-care industry. It is producing more drugs every year and spending millions of dollars to convince us that we need them. We are taking more drugs than ever before, but we aren't healthier. The evidence and effectiveness behind drug therapies can easily be manufactured, while the risks are downplayed. Many cancer patients are not told enough about the side effects of treatment and have no idea what they are in for when they agree to it. And the collateral damage can be lethal. The risk that chemotherapy and radiotherapy can make cancer more aggressive or cause more cancer in the body is rarely explained.

The tragedy is that even with the overwhelming evidence that conventional treatments don't cure most metastatic cancers, the pharmaceutical and medical industries have shown little interest in abandoning these destructive treatments. Instead they see it as an opportunity to create more drugs they can sell in conjunction with chemotherapy, in an attempt to make chemo work a little better or lessen its side effects. More drug therapies equal billions more in profits, regardless of curing the disease or saving the patient.

IT'S NOT LIKE I NEED YOUR BUSINESS

*It is difficult to get a man to understand something when
his salary depends upon his not understanding it.*

— UPTON SINCLAIR

DURING WORLD WAR I autopsies revealed that soldiers exposed
to the chemical warfare agent mustard gas had very low white
blood cell counts and depleted lymph nodes because of the effect
the poison had on their bone marrow. It was then theorized that
a mustard gas derivative might slow down the growth of certain
types of cancer cells. In 1943, pharmacologists Louis Goodman
and Alfred Gilman, along with thoracic surgeon Gustaf Lindskog,
injected nitrogen mustard into six terminal cancer patients. Two
of the patients with lymphosarcoma had "significant" but temporary tumor shrinkage, which had never been seen before. The
patients were not cured and eventually died. This led to another
series of experiments on approximately 150 patients. Some of
these patients with Hodgkin's disease, leukemia, and lymphosarcoma also had tumor shrinkage, but again none were cured.[1]

When the war was over, the results of these studies showing tumor shrinkage were published and the multibillion-dollar chemotherapy industry was born. Chemotherapy literally means "treating disease with chemicals." Nitrogen mustard was banned for use as a weapon under the 1993 Chemical Weapons Convention. It is still used today, however, decades later, in the form of several cancer drugs: cyclophosphamide, chlorambucil, ifosfamide, melphalan, and mechlorethamine, aka Mustargen. Here's what the manufacturer Merck has to say about Mustargen, as per the FDA website:

> Therapy with alkylating agents such as Mustargen may be associated with an increased incidence of a second malignant tumor, especially when such therapy is combined with other antineoplastic agents or radiation therapy.

CANCER IS BIG BUSINESS

Over $40 billion is spent every year on cancer drugs around the world. Cancer drugs are the second-largest category of pharmaceutical sales in the United States, after heart disease drugs, and are growing twice as fast as the rest of the market. Treating cancer is not a humanitarian pursuit; it is a billion-dollar business.

After eight years of undergrad and medical school, the average graduate ends up with about $150,000 in student loan debt. Their next step is three to five years of residency, which typically pays about $50,000 to $60,000 per year. After roughly 12 years of education and training, an oncologist can finally begin their career. It takes another five to ten years before they see firsthand that the cancer treatment methods they were taught in med school don't produce permanent remission for metastatic cancers, and that most of these patients do not survive. According to the 2017 Medscape Physician Compensation Report, oncologists make $330,000 per year on average yet only 57 percent of those surveyed felt "fairly compensated."

The oncology business model is different from other branches of medicine because you can't buy most chemotherapy drugs at your local pharmacy. Hospitals and oncology clinics buy cancer drugs at wholesale prices and then mark them up and sell them to you, charging you for the privilege of putting them in your body. Private practice oncologists make up to two-thirds of their income on the profit from chemo drugs.[2] This conflict of interest and legal profiting on drugs, known as a "buy and bill scheme," is unique to the cancer treatment world.

In 2003 in an attempt to reduce the financial incentives attached to drug therapies and clean up the seedy side of cancer treatment, Congress passed the Medicare Prescription Drug, Improvement, and Modernization Act, capping the markup on cancer drugs at 6 percent plus an administration fee. Consequently, oncologists began prescribing drugs with higher profit margins and increasing the number of treatments given to patients.[3] More expensive drugs plus more office visits equal more money.

The financial incentives aren't limited to drug therapies for cancer. As I mentioned in Chapter 4, the use of CT scans has increased from 1 million per year to about 80 million per year in the last 30 years. A 2013 study published in *The New England Journal of Medicine* found that urologists who owned their own radiotherapy equipment prescribed radiation three times as much as urologists who did not. The 10-year survival rate for all types of prostate cancer is about 98 percent because it's typically very slow growing, but doctors who own their own equipment were found to be treating 80-year-old men just as aggressively as young men.[4] According to Jean Mitchell, author of the report and professor at Georgetown University:

> It's crazy the way the system is set up. The patients are going to do what their physician tells them to do. The patient becomes almost like an ATM machine, with the doctor extracting as much revenue as they can.

In 2014 UnitedHealth Group published a study in which they paid oncologists in five medical groups a flat-rate payment per patient instead of paying them for each drug or service they provided. As a result the cost of cancer care in these groups fell by 34 percent over three years, saving patients $33 million.[5] When you remove the financial incentives, it changes the way oncologists treat patients.

INSIDE THE FDA

Nutrition and natural remedies have been used for centuries to support the body in healing, and many herbal medicinal formulas have been passed down from one generation to the next. Along the way, entrepreneurial types have bottled and sold all manner of tonics, lotions, and potions with curative claims. The FDA was established in 1902 to regulate the safety of ingredients in the food and drug industry and to limit the health claims that a manufacturer of medicine could make. Many popular "health tonics" sold before the FDA was established contained dangerous and highly addictive ingredients.

In the late 1800s, a small Atlanta company developed an elixir that they marketed as a "brain tonic" and pain reliever. The original formula contained cocaine from the coca leaf and caffeine from the African kola nut. It was sweet and fizzy and made you feel really, really good. In 1903, after 17 years of distribution, Coca-Cola removed the active cocaine from its formula and eventually stopped making health claims. Today the FDA requires extensive clinical trials before a drug or medicine is approved for medical use to treat a specific disease. The goal of the FDA approval process is to determine whether a drug is safe and effective, but a lot of inside money influences the approval of new drugs because of the enormous cost of drug development and clinical trials. One of those costs is the $2.1 million "user fee" that drug companies pay to the FDA each time they submit a new drug application for approval.

According to the Tufts Center for the Study of Drug Development, the average out-of-pocket cost to take a new drug from inception all the way to FDA approval is $1.3 billion. But that's only an average of the costs of the drugs that got FDA approval. It doesn't count all the money the drug companies spent researching and developing drugs that failed to get approval.

Forbes writer Matthew Herper totaled R & D spending from the 12 leading pharmaceutical companies from 1997 to 2011 and found that they had spent $802 billion to gain approval for 139 drugs, at an astounding average cost of $5.8 billion per drug.[6] Each new drug has the potential to make tens of billions of dollars in profit. With that much money at stake, it's not surprising that pharmaceutical companies try to influence the drug approval process in any way they can, including putting their own people on the FDA approval panels.

In October 2005 the renowned science journal *Nature* published an investigation of panels that write the clinical guidelines governing the diagnosis and treatment of patients with new drugs. They discovered that more than one-third of these authors declared financial links to relevant drug companies, with around 70 percent of panels being affected. In one case, every member of the panel had been paid by the company responsible for the drug that was ultimately recommended.[7]

Once the FDA approves new medications, drug company sales reps push them to doctors, who then prescribe them to you. If a significant number of patients die or suffer severe health problems caused by the drug, the FDA will eventually recall the dangerous medication. In most cases the manufacturer of the recalled drug has already made astronomical profits—enough to settle lawsuits for the permanent injuries and death that their drugs caused before they were recalled. Unless it's a vaccine. In that case, the U.S. government uses your tax dollars to settle the claims because the pharmaceutical industry has immunity from vaccine injury lawsuits. You can thank the National Childhood Vaccine Injury Act of 1986 for that.

Every drug medication available in the U.S. is a result of a cost-benefit analysis of its therapeutic value versus its harmful effects. Unfortunately, the behind-the-scenes process by which the FDA approves drugs, as well as the influence that pharmaceutical companies exert on the process, is not understood by the public. What may be the most surprising is that the FDA does not actually conduct its own independent drug safety testing. This research is done by the very companies who make the drugs. *PLoS Medicine* reported in 2013 that as many as half of all clinical trials are not published.[8]

Here are a few examples of "evidence-based," FDA-approved drugs that have been recalled in recent years. Painkiller Vioxx, taken by over 80 million people, was recalled for doubling heart attack risk if taken for 18 months or longer. In its promotional efforts, Merck created a fake scientific journal that contained ghost-written articles promoting Vioxx, which was marketed to doctors.[9] According to testimony in a Vioxx class action case in Australia, Merck also created a hit list to "destroy," "neutralize," or "discredit" doctors who spoke out against the irritable bowel syndrome drug Zelnorm, which was recalled due to eightfold increase in risk of heart attacks.[10] Diet drug Redux was recalled for a twenty-three-fold increase in the risk of primary pulmonary hypertension—abnormally high blood pressure in the arteries of the lungs that causes significant strain on the heart—after only three months on the drug.

CANCER CENTERS ARE COMPETING FOR YOUR BUSINESS

From 2005 to 2014, the amount of money spent on advertising by cancer treatment centers tripled. In 2014 alone 890 cancer centers spent $173 million on ads and over half of that was spent by Cancer Treatment Centers of America.[11] The majority of TV and magazine ads for U.S. cancer centers use emotional appeals rather than facts, leading to unrealistic expectations about treatment. A recent review of 409 television and magazine ads for 102 cancer centers found that 85 percent of ads used potentially misleading emotional appeals that seemed to equate treatment with cure.[12] Sixty-one percent of ads featured messages evoking hope for survival. Over half the ads included patient testimonials. Forty-one percent of ads described cancer treatment as a fight or battle, and a third of the ads were categorized by the study authors as "fear inducing."

Twenty-seven percent of cancer center ads promoted the benefits of cancer therapies, but none of the ads cited specific data to support their claims. Only 5 percent of ads mentioned costs and only 2 percent of ads gave objective information on treatment or talked about the typical results and risks such as physical suffering, financial hardship, cancer recurrence, and likelihood of eventual death.

Cancer center television ads often feature images of bald women and children accompanied by dramatic orchestral music, followed by witty taglines like "Fighters Wanted" or "Making Cancer History." The study authors suggested that cancer center ads that evoke emotions of fear and hope may mislead patients and their families to pursue treatments that are either unnecessary or unsupported by scientific evidence.

CANCER TREATMENTS DESTROY HEALTH AND WEALTH

One often unanticipated side effect of cancer treatment is its "financial toxicity." For most patients, the cancer treatment conveyor belt involves countless office visits, blood tests, CT and PET scans, surgical procedures, radiation therapy, chemotherapy, additional drugs for the side effects of treatments, emergency room visits, hospital stays, physical therapy, and cosmetic procedures like breast reconstruction, custom wigs, and nipple tattoos. It all adds up to a ton of money. In 2012, 11 of the 12 cancer drugs approved by the FDA were priced at over $100,000 per year. That same year physicians at Memorial Sloan Kettering Cancer Center took a stand and refused to prescribe colon cancer drug Zaltrap because it cost over $11,000 per month and was not shown to work any better than Avastin, which only cost $5,000 per month. As a result, the manufacturer of Zaltrap came down on the price. These conscientious doctors deserve kudos for standing up to Big Pharma, but unfortunately, since then, new drugs are more expensive than ever.

Cancer treatment can be financially devastating for someone who doesn't have insurance, but even those covered by insurance can end up bankrupt. The total cost of cancer treatment can range from several hundred thousand dollars to well over a million, and it's not uncommon for a cancer patient's medical debt to range from tens of thousands of dollars to over six figures. The financial problem is compounded when many cancer patients find themselves unable to work, often not because of the cancer but because of the brutal debilitating treatments they are told they must endure to increase their chances of survival, or to maybe live just a little longer.

A comprehensive study on cancer patients in Washington state diagnosed between 1995 and 2009 reported that they were two and half times more likely to go bankrupt than anyone else, and younger cancer patients were two to five times more likely to go bankrupt than patients over 65.[13] According to the 2004 Medical Expenditure Panel Survey, $130 million is spent out of pocket every year by cancer patients not on Medicare. Patients and their families are draining their life savings, mortgaging their houses, borrowing from friends, maxing out their credit cards, and begging for money from anyone who will give, with the hopes that another round of treatments might cure them or buy them more time. After suffering through months, even years of brutal therapies, many cancer patients find themselves dropped off at the end of the line, broke or bankrupt, with irreversible damage done to their bodies and little time left to live.

THE CATCH-22 OF CANCER TREATMENT

Both chemotherapy and radiation are capable of shrinking tumors and reducing cancer in the short term, but in many cases, the cancer comes back more aggressively than before and the patient is then subjected to more aggressive treatments. Thus begins the downward spiral. Endless rounds of chemo and radiation treatments may keep the cancer under control for a while but destroy the patient in the process. The unfortunate and all too common end result is that the cancer eventually becomes resistant to all treatments, at which point either hospice is suggested or, as a last-ditch effort, the patient is given the opportunity to be a guinea pig in an experimental clinical trial, a practice known inside the industry as "desperation oncology."

At this point, many cancer patients are devastated, discouraged, tired of suffering, and too broke to try anything else. Many are depressed and hopeless, and lose the will to live. The few who still have a strong desire to live after doctors have told them, "We've done everything we can" often begin looking into natural, nontoxic, and alternative therapies as a last-ditch effort. Despite having the odds stacked against them, I have met many terminal cancer patients who have healed themselves after doctors sent them home to die. There is always hope!

THE ELEPHANT
IN THE WAITING ROOM

Men occasionally stumble over the truth,
but most of them pick themselves up and hurry off
as if nothing ever happened.

— WINSTON CHURCHILL

I stood in line for an hour and fifteen minutes for the Dumbo ride.
After a minute I was like, I'm the Dumbo.

— JIM GAFFIGAN

TODAY IN THE UNITED STATES, 1 in 537 people die from cancer, with an annual death toll of over 580,000. Every day over 6,000 people are diagnosed with cancer and roughly 1,500 people die of the disease. More people are dying from cancer each year than in all of the U.S. wars combined, and cancer is now the number one killer in the world with an annual death toll of about 7.6 million people. Nearly half of American men and a third of American women are expected to get cancer in their lifetime.

At the turn of the 20th century, cancer was killing 1 in 1,500 Americans. By the 1950s, the cancer death rate had tripled and chemotherapy was introduced. Twenty years later, President Nixon declared "War on Cancer" with the passage of the National Cancer Act of 1971. Since then over $500 billion American tax dollars (adjusted for inflation) have been spent on research for promising new treatments. Undeterred by the "war," the cancer death rate continued to climb and peaked at 215 deaths per 100,000 people in 1991. It has declined since then, but the reason for this decline has very little to do with improvements in cancer treatment.

Brace yourself for the most shocking statistic in all of Cancerdom. Since the introduction of chemotherapy in the 1950s, the overall cancer death rate in the United States has only improved by 5 percent. And that includes an adjustment for age and population size. The death rate is the purest measure of progress and we've barely made any in 60 years. To give credit where it is due, the most notable progress has been made in curatively treating a handful of cancers like chronic myeloid leukemia, Hodgkin's and non-Hodgkin's lymphoma, testicular cancer, and childhood leukemia, many of which have an average 10-year survival rate between 80 and 90 percent. The cancer industry frequently highlights these exceptions, but treatments for epithelial cancers (solid tumor carcinomas), which make up about 80 percent of all cancers, have made little to no progress in lowering the death rate. So why is this lack of improvement so at odds with what we hear from the medical industry about our progress in the war on cancer?

In 2016 the American Cancer Society, which receives funding from drug companies including Merck, Pfizer, Eli Lilly, AstraZeneca, and Genentech, released a report celebrating the fact that the cancer death rate had dropped 23 percent from its peak in 1991 and claiming that 1.7 million deaths have been avoided. This blurb circled the globe and was lauded by the media as "significant progress in the war on cancer due to increased screening, early detection and better treatments." But that doesn't tell the whole story.

THE SMOKING GUN

The real cause for the 23 percent improvement in the overall cancer death rate since 1991 is largely attributed to the reduction in cigarette smoking, and to a lesser extent the reduction in hormone replacement therapy (HRT) for women. Smoking is the number one cause of cancer, and lung cancer is our number one cancer killer. Eighty-three percent of lung cancer patients die within five years of diagnosis. Conservative estimates indicate that the reduction in smoking is responsible for 40 percent of the decrease in male cancer deaths from 1991 to 2003.[1] This 40 percent drop in the death rate of our number one cancer killer had a huge impact on the overall cancer death rate, but somehow "early detection and innovations in cancer treatment" got most of the credit in the headlines.

Another factor that contributed to the drop in the overall cancer death rate is that women are taking fewer prescription drugs that cause cancer. In 2002 the Women's Health Initiative reported an increased risk of breast cancer, heart attacks, and strokes among women taking Prempro, an HRT that combined estrogen and progestin. In the following year, HRT prescriptions dropped sharply. In 2001 61 million HRT prescriptions were written. By 2004 the number of HRT prescriptions had dropped by two-thirds to 21 million. In that same period of time, new breast cancer diagnosis rates dropped by 8.6 percent.[2]

A 2015 analysis of 52 studies suggested an association between short-term use of HRT during menopause and a 40 percent increased relative risk of developing ovarian cancer. This risk declines after stopping treatment, but women who used HRT for 5 years or more were found to have increased risk even after 10 years.[3]

PHANTOM SURVIVORS

According to the National Cancer Institute's Surveillance, Epidemiology, and End Results (SEER) data, the overall five-year survival rate for all cancers combined has improved about 40 percent since 1975. This improvement in five-year survival, the standard by which the effectiveness of cancer treatment is measured, looks phenomenal on paper but often means very little in the real world of cancer patients.

Oftentimes five-year survival statistics do not distinguish between disease-free survival (DFS) and those who are alive with disease (AWD). If a woman is diagnosed with breast cancer and is alive five years later, she is counted as a successful five-year survivor. If she still has cancer, she is still a success. If she is an invalid, bedridden, unable to feed herself, or on life support, she is still a success. If she dies five years and one month after diagnosis, she is still a success. But if during those five years she dies from one of the various side effects of cancer treatment like a surgical complication, a hospital-acquired infection, a drug reaction, chemo toxicity, or organ failure, she may not be counted at all if she didn't technically die from "cancer."

Here's how misleading and biased five-year survival statistics can be. If 10 women are diagnosed with late-stage breast cancer at age 60 and all die by age 64, their five-year survival rate is 0 percent. If these same women are diagnosed with cancer earlier at age 58 and all die by 64, their five-year survival is now 100 percent. Increased screening and early detection made a remarkable improvement in their five-year survival, but they are all still dead at 64. That statistical phenomenon is known as lead-time bias. Surprisingly, your doctor may have no idea what lead-time bias is or how it has inflated survival statistics. In one study, 54 of 65 physicians surveyed did not understand lead-time bias. Of the 11 physicians who indicated they did, only two explained it correctly.[4]

Many cancer patients are not actually living longer due to improved cancer treatments; they are just finding out sooner that they have cancer, thanks to early detection. In addition, early stage cancers that are not life threatening and may spontaneously regress (heal) without treatment are also being counted and treated with lumpectomies, mastectomies, radiation, and chemo. One example is ductal carcinoma in situ (DCIS), also known as stage 0 breast cancer, which accounts for 20 to 30 percent of all breast cancer diagnoses and has a nearly 100 percent 10-year survival rate. A study of more than 100,000 women with DCIS found that their risk of dying of breast cancer was the same as women with no signs of breast cancer. Thanks to current guidelines, 20 to 30 out of every 100 breast cancer patients are being unnecessarily diagnosed and treated for something that isn't cancer.[5] Just like lead-time bias, overdiagnosis bias has made huge improvements on five-year survival rates and virtually no improvement on cancer death rates.

The elephant in the waiting room is that the cancer industry isn't curing most cancers. The fact that the overall cancer death rate has barely improved in 60 years, while the cancer industry continues to tout dubious 5-year survival rates and take credit for the reduction in cancer deaths from less smoking, is a powerful indictment against this institution. There's simply no other logical explanation for the spinning of statistics on such a grand scale. Meanwhile, the cancer industry continues the widespread practice of "finding and successfully treating" cancers that would never have been life threatening, while simultaneously failing to cure the cancers that are. If winning the war on cancer means curing the disease, the cancer industry is most definitely losing. In the meantime, the cancer industry is generating over $100 billion in revenue per year. Losing has never been more lucrative.

As frustrating as the overdiagnosis and overtreatment problem is, the tide is turning. The use of chemotherapy to treat early stage breast cancer is on the decline. A study of roughly 3,000 women with early stage breast cancer—and some 500 doctors who treated them—found that use of chemotherapy declined overall from 34.5 percent of cases in 2013 to 21.3 percent of cases in 2015.[6]

A significant advance occurred in August 2016 when the results of the MINDACT phase 3 clinical trial were published confirming that nearly half of early stage breast cancer patients have been receiving unnecessary treatments. The trial used a genetic test called MammaPrint to determine a patient's risk of breast cancer recurrence after surgery. Use of the test reduced chemotherapy treatment by 46 percent among the over 3,300 patients in the trial categorized as having a high risk of breast cancer recurrence based on current treatment criteria. The "high risk" patients with a low risk MammaPrint score who did not do chemo had a 95 percent five-year distant metastasis free survival rate.[7]

You now know vastly more about the cancer industry than I did when I decided to take control of my health and start my healing journey. Back in January 2004, I had one book with one cancer healing testimony and very little scientific evidence to substantiate the author's claims. Even so, the message of radical life change to get to the root cause of disease and restore health resonated with me, and in the absence of verifiable facts, I made my decision based on instincts, intuition, and faith.

Despite my critical view of the cancer industry, I am not anti-doctor or anti-chemo. I am pro-life, pro-health, and pro-healing. Any strategy or therapy that promotes health and healing is one worth pursuing. Any therapy that is destructive, threatens to do more harm than good, and has little evidence of long-term success is one that should be approached with caution and considered carefully.

Although I've highlighted many of the perils, pitfalls, and failures of the conventional cancer industry, my intention is not to talk you out of conventional treatment. Rather, it is to equip you with knowledge to make an informed decision, the best decision for you. And hopefully to spur you on to continue researching and educating yourself. In the following chapters I will show you what I did and what my radical life transformation looked like.

THE BEAT CANCER MINDSET

Luck is not a factor.
Hope is not a strategy.
Fear is not an option.

— JAMES CAMERON

Whether you believe you can do a thing or not,
you are right.

— HENRY FORD

IN THE FIRST YEAR OF MY HEALING JOURNEY, one of the physical therapies I employed, along with chiropractic adjustments and acupuncture, was a form of therapeutic massage called structural integration, also known as "Rolfing." Three months after my diagnosis, I went to see a structural integration practitioner named Elinor. During our first meeting, she asked me a series of questions, the last of which was surprising and slightly terrifying. She said, "Before we get started, I need to know if you really want to live."

Like many cancer patients, I had mainly been focused on not dying. No one had ever asked me if I actually wanted to live. Isn't that a given? Doesn't everybody want to live?

Did I really want to live? For a brief moment, I feared that maybe deep down I didn't, that perhaps, subconsciously, I had a death wish. So I asked myself, *Do I want to live? Do I?* I searched my heart. At first I didn't know what the answer was. Despite my ambition and the confidence I outwardly projected, I had never really liked myself. I was afraid that secretly maybe I didn't want to live and that maybe my cancer was the manifestation of years of painful insecurity and mental and emotional self-sabotage. But in that moment, I realized that even if that was true, I could confront those thoughts and feelings and behavior. I could change.

"Yes. I want to live."

If you've been diagnosed with a terminal illness, this is the most powerful question you can ask yourself. So go ahead, ask yourself, "Do I want to live?" If your answer is yes, my next question for you is "Why?" Why do you want to live? If you are not sure, take a few minutes to think about what you have to live for. Your reasons to live might be people in your life who need you, people you want to love and serve. Your reason might be a purpose, a calling, a mission you haven't accomplished, a dream you haven't fulfilled, or it might be all of the above. Write down or type up the list of your reasons to live and put this list in places where you will see it every day. Tack the list on the wall. Write it in lipstick on your bathroom mirror. Make it the background on your computer screen. Take a picture and make it the lock screen on your phone. Keep your reasons to live in front of you and on your mind throughout the day every day.

I had several strong reasons to live. First and foremost I wanted to live for my wife and for my parents. At the time of my diagnosis, Micah and I had been together for eight years (dated for six, married for two). I couldn't bear the thought of leaving her a widow. Equally painful was the thought of my parents standing beside her at my graveside, burying me, their only child. Beyond that I had dreams and aspirations. I wanted to live a long, full life. I had an entrepreneurial spirit, and I wanted to build a successful business. I wanted to have children and grandchildren, and maybe even meet my great-grandchildren. I wanted to have adventures and travel the world. I wanted to serve the purpose of God in my generation.

Healing cancer starts in your mind and your heart, and with a choice. The choice to live.

Some cancer patients don't have a strong will to live. They may be satisfied with what they've accomplished in life and are ready to die. If this is you, that's okay! What I would like to encourage you to do is to help the people around you understand that you are ready to die so they won't continue to pressure you into doing things you don't want to do. If you don't want to do treatment, don't do it. This is your life and you should do what you want to do. You should make the most of the time you have left and live your life to the fullest. Spend time with people you love. Make your bucket list and start checking it off.

In January 2012 my cousin Jeff was diagnosed with stage IV colon cancer. He was told that he would only live for about six months without chemo but that he could live up to two years if he did treatment. He accepted his prognosis and agreed to the treatments that his doctors said would "buy him more time" but would not cure him. He set up a CaringBridge page and chronicled his journey through cancer treatment, which showed his inspiring strength and courage. In one e-mail to family, he mentioned that he hoped to be able run one more marathon between chemo treatments, but the tone of his e-mails suggested that he had accepted that he would not be cured. During this time his mother was strongly encouraging him to get a second opinion and to consider incorporating nutrition and nontoxic therapies as I did. She begged him to talk to me and I reached out to him via e-mail, but he did not respond. Later he told his mother in another e-mail that he and I were very different and that he didn't buy into fads or self-help books.

After surgery to remove the tumor in his colon, Jeff felt better and was in good spirits, but within a few weeks after starting chemo his health took a dramatic turn for the worse as the tumors grew rapidly in his abdomen and liver. He could not eat or even keep water down, and he told the doctors that if living meant continuing to be in the condition he was in—i.e., not being able to eat or drink—he did not want to live and would just let the cancer take him, and he hoped it would be quick. Jeff was gone in about three months after diagnosis, just after his 49th birthday.

THE BEAT CANCER MINDSET

As I've thought about my cousin's cancer experience and reflected on the path he chose, I've come to realize that he was right. He and I are different. Introspection does not come naturally to me, but as I began teaching others about health, nutrition, healing, and survival, I was often asked why I made the decisions I made, and I was forced to self-analyze. I realized what made me different; it was the mindset I adopted, which was born out of my determination to get well and to live. Since I started my journey, I've read about, met, and interviewed many people who have healed all types and stages of cancer, and I've seen that same mindset in every single one of them. I call it the Beat Cancer Mindset. This mindset is the single most important factor, the linchpin in every successful healing story.

The Beat Cancer Mindset has five components:

➤ Accept total responsibility for your health.

➤ Be willing to do whatever it takes.

➤ Take massive action.

➤ Make plans for the future.

➤ Enjoy your life and the process.

1) Accept total responsibility for your health.

The first question on a cancer patient's mind after diagnosis is "Why did this happen to me? How did I get cancer?" The revelation I had in January 2004 was that the way I was living was killing me. If you have cancer, I believe you should assume the same. My intention is not to blame you or shame you but to empower you to take control of your situation and change your life. Many of the cancer-causing factors in your life can be removed and your risk of getting a recurrence or dying from cancer can be greatly reduced, just by your choices. Your choices matter.

People who care about you are going to tell you the truth. Sometimes the truth stings a little, but the truth will set you free. Accepting responsibility for your health starts with considering the possibility that cancer may be your fault. Maybe some bad decisions, bad habits, or ignorance over the course of your life contributed to your cancer. I know mine did. There's no need to beat yourself up about it or wallow in guilt, self-pity, or regret. Instead now is the time to evaluate your life, accept whatever part you played, and learn from your mistakes. Now is the time to identify the cancer causers in your life, radically change, and move forward.

One of the most troubling things I've ever heard a cancer patient say is, "I'm not going to let cancer change me." On the surface, this proclamation of defiance to the disease gives the impression of strength, determination, and willpower and could easily serve as a rallying cry for cancer fighters, but tragically, it is denial and disempowerment in disguise. It was denial that she had contributed in any way to her situation, and it was an acknowledgment that she did not believe she had the power to affect her health and her future. She did not survive. And the gravity of her statement still haunts me. Denial is far more dangerous than blaming yourself. Accepting the blame is taking responsibility. Taking responsibility for your circumstance empowers you to take control of your life and to change for the better.

Every day in cancer clinics all over the world, patients are told that their cancer is probably the result of bad luck or bad genes. This turns patients into victims. The logic is simple: nothing you did caused or contributed to your disease; therefore, there is nothing you can do to reverse it. If you have family history, they may tell you it's genetic. If you don't have any family history, they may still tell you it's genetic. Heredity and genetics are easy scapegoats, but fewer than 5 percent of cancers are genetic, and not everyone with a "cancer gene" develops cancer. Genes may load the gun, but your diet, lifestyle, and environment pull the trigger. However, if you believe that you are powerless and that there is nothing you can do to positively affect your health and your future, your only hope is medical procedures and pharmaceutical drugs.

You are not powerless and you are not a victim. The health or disease you are experiencing today is largely the result of the diet and lifestyle decisions you've made in the past. If you abuse your body, it is going to break down sooner, but if you take care of your body it will work better and you will increase your odds of health, healing, and long life. Today's choices affect tomorrow's health. Your choices matter!

Cancer is not the cause of a sick body. It is the effect of a sick body. You aren't sick because you have cancer—you have cancer because you are sick. When you accept that you may have played a part in your body becoming vulnerable to developing cancer, you will also realize that you can play a part in healing it. If you broke it, maybe you can fix it. If you caused it, maybe you can cure it. If the way you were living resulted in disease, maybe changing the way you live will result in health. Early in my cancer journey, I realized that I had never really taken care of myself. Being thin I assumed I had a free pass to eat whatever I wanted, and for many years I was unknowingly poisoning and polluting my body. I was living on processed food, fast food, and junk food. I was well fed but nutrient deficient. I was stuffed but starving. I had a history of exposure to environmental toxins. And I had a lot of unhealthy stress and negative emotions in my life. Deep down I hated myself, and I was desperately seeking the attention and approval of others to combat my insecurity and unhappiness. All of these factors contributed to my disease. And they all had to do with my choices. I needed to change, and cancer was the divine tap on the shoulder, the catalyst for that change.

2) Be willing to do whatever it takes.

Once you have accepted responsibility for your health, the next step is being willing to do whatever it takes to get well, which means being willing to turn your life upside down, to change everything. If restoring my health meant getting as close to nature as possible by sleeping in the woods in a tent, I was willing to do it. If it meant trekking out into the wilderness for a 40-day water fast like Jesus, I was willing to do it. Fortunately I didn't have to resort to either of those two things, but they were on my radar. I became a detective, determined to identify and eliminate anything in my life that may have contributed to my disease. I stopped eating to satisfy my appetite and sensual cravings and began eating to feed my cells, restore my health, and save my life. I wasn't living to eat anymore; I was eating to live.

Most cancer patients have a strong will to live in the beginning, but unfortunately most of them have also been convinced that "doing whatever it takes," "living strong," and "fighting cancer" just mean suffering through brutal and destructive cancer treatments. Whether you do conventional treatments or not, the Beat Cancer Mindset means taking an active role in your health and healing, not solely relying on someone else to cure you. I radically changed my diet and lifestyle. I gave up all the unhealthy food I loved to eat. I did every natural, nontoxic therapy I could find and afford. I faced my fears, admitted my faults, changed the way I thought, reached out to God and asked for help, and forgave everyone who had hurt me. This was a lot more work than showing up for chemo and having my doctor's permission to eat burgers, ice cream, and pizza, and not changing my life, but I knew I had to do it.

The difference between successful people and unsuccessful people is not motivation. Motivation is unpredictable and unreliable. It is easy to be motivated when you've started something new and exciting, but when the excitement wears off so does the motivation, and lack of motivation becomes an excuse for inaction. What keeps people going when their motivation is low is determination. Determination is the force inside you that cannot be stopped, even when the storms of life come against you. Determination is doing what you know needs to be done, whether or not you feel like it at the time.

During this process I became acutely aware of the spirit-mind-body connection as it relates to health and realized that not only did I need to change my diet and lifestyle, but I also needed to change the way I was thinking.

My perspective on cancer is different from most. I don't see cancer as something to be fought or killed; I see it as something to be healed. There is a battle involved in healing cancer, but it's not so much a battle in the body as it is a battle in the mind. In order to heal your body, you must first win the battle in your mind. *Changing your thoughts will change your life.*

But first you have to stop lying to yourself. You have to stop making excuses and stop making bad decisions that sabotage your life and your health. And this starts with changing your thoughts.

Instead of dwelling on negativity, feeling sorry for myself, being jealous of everyone who didn't have cancer, worrying about my future, and allowing depression and discouragement to paralyze me, I took control of my thoughts and chose to think of myself the way I wanted to be. *I am healed. I am healthy. I am well. I am going to live.* That Beat Cancer Mindset prompted me to take massive action every day to promote health and healing in my body.

Did these thoughts come naturally? Absolutely not. I had to choose to think that way every single day. Worry was not an option. Failure (death) was not an option. I had to succeed, and I had to live. I realized that my mind was like a track on repeat, playing the same negative thoughts over and over again. I had to reprogram my mind. When I caught myself thinking negatively, I chose to think positively. I chose to speak life out of my mouth and not allow outside influences, fear, and doubt to sway me. When you think and speak this way, you empower your creative subconscious mind to assist you in the process, and you find supernatural strength to do things you never thought you could.

Your conscious mind and subconscious mind are powerful. Your beliefs are powerful. Patients who believe treatment will help them often respond better than those who don't. The placebo effect is real. In my experience patients who go through the motions of treatment and therapies to appease those around them but don't believe they can get well rarely do. They subliminally sabotage the process and often make impulsive, irrational, emotion-based decisions that are not conducive to healing.

When a doctor tells a patient they are going to die in a matter of months, it can become a self-fulfilling prophecy. They often lose all hope and stop trying to live. They believe they are going to die and they usually do, as predicted. This is eerily not unlike a hex or a curse. No doctor has the authority to dictate the end of your life unless you give it to them. They do not know when you will die. They are just lumping you into a statistical group based on your age, cancer type, stage, and other factors. Your thoughts and beliefs create your life, your health, and your future. And when faced with a terminal prognosis, you have a choice of how to process that information. You can choose to believe it, or you can choose to reject it and become determined to prove your doctor wrong. It's okay to accept a diagnosis, assuming it has been validated by several sources, but you don't have to accept a prognosis that you're going to die in a certain amount of time because a doctor or a statistic said so. Defy the odds and be the exception. That's the Beat Cancer Mindset.

3) Take massive action.

The third characteristic of successful survivors is massive action. Minimal action typically produces minimal results, but massive action produces massive results. Massive Action is radical action. It's going against the grain. It's swimming upstream when everyone else is floating downstream. It's action that draws jealousy and criticism from others. Humans by nature are resistant to change and tend to have a "crab mentality." If you put crabs in a bucket and one tries to escape, the other crabs will pull it back down. In the same way, people often pull each other down out of envy, spite, or competitiveness. Massive Action may appear crazy to people around you and they may try to talk you out of it, like they did me, but don't let them.

Massive Action is facing your flaws, faults, and fears, changing your whole life, getting rid of everything that might be keeping you sick, and replacing disease promoters with health promoters. Sometimes small changes can produce big results. I love when that happens. But if that's what you're hoping for, your hope is in the wrong place because your hope is for a quick fix. That's not the Beat Cancer Mindset. That's the Magic Bullet Mindset. And the conventional and alternative cancer industries are both full of people ready to take advantage of anyone looking for a shortcut. You didn't get cancer overnight and you aren't going to get rid of it overnight. There is no miracle cure or magic bullet. Long-term healing requires massive action and a total life change. *Point your ship toward Healthy Island and stay the course.*

I've seen many cancer patients experience dramatic turnarounds in their health and have tumors shrink and even disappear in as little as 30 to 90 days using nutrition and nontoxic therapies, but I've also seen some of them become lazy and complacent and slide back into their old unhealthy habits. Then the cancer comes back. The first two years after a cancer diagnosis are the most critical. This is when cancer is most likely to return or spread. Two years of hard-core healthy living is an ideal short-term target, and beyond that, in order to stay healthy long term, you have to make your health a priority for life. Every day of your life is a page in your story. Your thoughts, decisions, and actions each day write your story. Take massive action to change your life and be 100 percent committed to the process. 100 percent is easy. 99 percent is hard.

4) Make plans for the future.

Document every detail of your cancer journey. Journal. Do a video diary. Plan on being well and document what you're doing so you can use what you've learned to help other people once you are well. You need a future goal to work toward, and making plans for the future is very important. The spirit-mind-body connection is a mystery, but something powerful happens when you plan for the future. You're planning to live. You're sending signals of life to your body. Don't be afraid to make plans for the future. I know the default response is, "Well, I don't know if I'll be here in a year or two years . . ." Instead of thinking that way, plan on living a long life. Sketch out your life goals, write down the things you want to accomplish, and keep those goals in front of you and start working toward them.

Making plans for the future is so important. When I was diagnosed, I didn't have children and I really wanted to have a family. I wanted to be a dad. The decision to start a family three months after being diagnosed was a huge risk, but it took my focus off cancer, strengthened my will to live, and brought a new dimension of purpose into my life. If Micah and I had agreed not to have children for fear of an unknown future, we would not have our two beautiful daughters, the greatest joys in our life.

5) Enjoy your life and the process.

Don't let fear and worry steal your joy. Make a decision to live in the present and to enjoy your life right now. Depression suppresses your immune system. If you're depressed, fearful, anxious, or worried, it makes you more vulnerable to cancer. Instead focus on things that bring you hope, optimism, encouragement, and joy. Start living your life, really living. There's an organization for young adult cancer patients called Stupid Cancer and I love their slogan, which is "Get Busy Living."

Now is the time to live. There are a thousand different ways you could die besides cancer. You could die in a car wreck. You could trip and hit your head on the pavement. You could choke on a peppermint. There's no point in letting cancer paralyze you into depression and inaction. Start doing things you've always wanted to do. Get out there. Live your life. Do fun stuff. Do some skydiving, mountain climbing, and bull riding like it says in the Tim McGraw song "Live Like You Were Dying." Make a commitment to enjoy your life and to enjoy the process. And Get Busy Living!

Even if some of these changes are difficult for you, like quitting smoking, giving up your favorite unhealthy foods, or eating vegetables you've never liked, you've got to keep your perspective because there are way worse things than vegetables. And when you get well, you can look back and know it was all worth it. This is a new chapter, a new season in life, a new adventure that should be dominated by gratitude. *Gratitude is the secret to happiness.*

Count your blessings every day. Don't focus on what you don't have. Focus on what you *do* have. Don't focus on what you can't do. Focus on what you *can* do. Cancer cut a dividing line in your life. If you're focused on the past, longing for the days before cancer and wishing things were the way they used to be, you will only make yourself more miserable. *What you focus on expands.*

Focus on joy, happiness, love, and gratitude and they will increase in your life. Focus on the present and on the things you can do today to improve your health and make your life better. In 2004 I was struggling to build a real estate business, barely making ends meet, and living in a tiny house, and I had cancer. I had every reason to be negative, bitter, and angry. But I learned how to exercise gratitude, how to be thankful, how to focus on all the good things in my life instead of the bad, and how to be happy in my most difficult season of life. And although I would rather not go through cancer again, I know with absolute certainty that what it taught me changed me for the better. The worst thing that ever happened to me has made my life more fulfilling than I could ever have imagined.

In the following chapters, I'm going to show you how to transform your life and how to take Massive Action to promote health and healing, which includes eliminating cancer causers, eating an evidence-based anti-cancer diet, and replacing your health-destroying habits with health-promoting ones. Finally, and most importantly, we'll talk about how to heal mentally, emotionally, and spiritually.

PLANTS VERSUS ZOMBIES

How Nutrition Fights Cancer

OVER 100,000 NUTRITIONAL SCIENCE STUDIES are published every year that demonstrate how naturally occurring compounds in plants can assist the body in preventing and reversing chronic disease. But because the pharmaceutical industry can't figure out how to extract most of the beneficial compounds in fruits, vegetables, herbs, and spices, synthesize them, and patent them for profit, this valuable research is largely ignored by the medical industry.

We've spent a lot of time talking about what you shouldn't put in your body and about how our Western diet promotes cancer. Now, as we begin to build your Massive Action Plan, we're going to talk about what you should put on your fork and into your body. In this chapter, we go deeper into the foods that fight cancer.

EATING TO BEAT CANCER

There are many different ways cancer can be stopped. Some compounds cause DNA damage, killing the cancer cell directly. Others cause apoptosis, which is programmed cell death, aka cancer cell suicide. Some are anti-proliferative; they stop cancer cells from spreading. Some compounds disrupt cancer cell metabolism. And others are anti-angiogenic. (Bet you can't say that last one five times fast.) We all have microscopic cancer cells in our bodies, but they can't grow into tumors any bigger than about 2 millimeters without first forming new blood vessels. This process is called angiogenesis, and blocking tumors from forming new blood vessels—a process known as anti-angiogenesis—is a very good thing. Avastin was the first anti-angiogenic drug approved by the FDA for cancer treatment but it is not a cure, has deadly side effects, and lost FDA approval for use in breast cancer. Fortunately there is a natural, nontoxic alternative: fruits and vegetables! Many phytonutrients in plant foods, such as apigenin and luteolin in parsley and celery, as well as fisetin in onions and strawberries, also have the ability to block the formation of new tumor blood vessels through anti-angiogenesis.

According to the research of Dr. William Li, president, medical director, and cofounder of the Angiogenesis Foundation, some of the most potent anti-angiogenic foods are green tea, ginseng, strawberries, blackberries, blueberries, raspberries, oranges, grapefruit, lemons, apples, pineapples, cherries, red grapes, kale, maitake mushrooms, turmeric, nutmeg, lavender, artichokes, pumpkins, parsley, garlic, tomatoes, olive oil, and even red wine and dark chocolate.[1] However, if you have cancer, I think it's a good idea to avoid alcohol until you are several years in the clear, as alcohol consumption can increase cancer risk. Dr. Li gave an excellent TED talk highlighting his discoveries in the field of nutrition and anti-angiogenesis called "Can We Eat to Starve Cancer?" And many of the foods I just listed aren't just anti-angiogenic. Like most plant foods, they contain compounds that cause cancer cell death, stop cancer from spreading, and disrupt cancer cell metabolism.

FRUIT VERSUS CANCER

Researchers at Cornell University conducted a study in which they dripped the freshly extracted juice of 11 common fruits on human liver cancer cells to see what would happen. Pineapples, pears, oranges, and peaches had very little effect on the liver cancer cells directly, but bananas and grapefruit cut the cancer cell growth by about 40 percent. Red grapes, strawberries, and apples were twice as potent as the bananas and grapefruit, but the tart fruits—cranberries and lemons—were the most powerful. Cranberries had the highest anti-cancer phenolic and antioxidant activity and cut liver cancer cell growth by 85 percent with only a third of the dose of apples and strawberries.[2] Lemons came in a close second. Researchers also noted that the higher the dose used, the more effective they were.

Cranberries have been shown to have anti-cancer effects on 17 different cancers in vitro and on 9 different cancers in animal studies, including cancers of the colon, bladder, esophagus, stomach, and prostate as well as lymphoma and glioblastoma.[3] In one study cranberries were fractionated in an attempt to isolate the active cancer-fighting compounds, but the isolated compounds did not work nearly as well as the whole fruit extract.[4] This is because the nutrients in whole foods are perfectly designed to work together synergistically to promote health in the body. The whole is greater than the sum of its parts, which is why many natural compounds don't translate to patented pharmaceutical medicine. In many cases they just don't work when isolated or altered in the lab. Anti-cancer nutrients are typically most potent when eaten in whole-food form, and the pharmaceutical and medical industries can't make any money selling lemons and cranberries to cancer patients.

Berries are the most potent anti-cancer fruits, partly due to their ability to protect and repair damage from oxidative stress and inflammation. Blueberries contain immune-boosting and anti-cancer compounds like ellagic acid, anthocyanins, and caffeic acid. One study reported that athletes who ate about two cups of blueberries per day for six weeks nearly doubled the amount of cancer-destroying natural killer cells in their blood from about 2 billion to 4 billion cells.[5] When eaten immediately before exercise, blueberries were also found to reduce oxidative stress and inflammation.

Raspberries, strawberries, and blackberries also contain ellagic acid and other compounds with anti-mutagenic effects that can protect your cells from free radicals and DNA damage, as well as slow down or stop cancer cell growth for many types of cancer. One laboratory study of berries versus cancer cells found that raspberry extract blocked cervical cancer cell growth by 50 percent. Strawberries blocked it by 75 percent.[6] Another study found organic strawberry extracts to be more potent and effective against colon and breast cancer cells than conventional strawberries.[7] In a 2011 randomized phase II clinical trial, researchers gave patients with precancerous esophageal lesions 60 grams of powdered freeze-dried strawberries every day for six months. At the end of six months, half the patients were disease free. The precancerous lesions were gone, and their tumor markers dropped dramatically, with just strawberries.[8] Another study found that black raspberries could stop the growth of precancerous oral lesions and even reverse cancer completely when patients applied black raspberries topically, simply spreading a black raspberry paste on the cancerous lesions in their mouth for six weeks.[9]

Lemons are everywhere and they're super cheap. Blueberries, blackberries, raspberries, and strawberries are also not hard to find, but cranberries present a few challenges. Fresh cranberries are not easy to find and even harder to eat because they are so tart. Store-bought cranberry juice is not an option because it's pasteurized, filtered, and often has sugar added. Dried cranberries, aka "craisins," are tasty, but they almost always have added processed sugar and oil, which could negate some of their beneficial effects. The best options are buying frozen organic cranberries at your local grocery store to blend into smoothies. You can also buy organic freeze-dried cranberry powder online and add it to juice or smoothies.

SUPERFOOD SPOTLIGHT: INDIAN GOOSEBERRY

Used for centuries in Indian ayurvedic medicine to treat nearly every condition known to man, and currently the top contender for the most incredible berry on earth, is amla, aka amalaki, the Indian gooseberry. Amla berries look like a cross between a green grape and a Ping-Pong ball and have the highest antioxidant content of any food known to man, with 200 times the antioxidant content of blueberries. Alma also has the second-highest concentration of vitamin C next to camu camu fruit. To put it in perspective, the average American meal has 25 to 100 units of antioxidants. One teaspoon of amla powder has nearly 800 units of antioxidants.

In a 2010 study, amla fruit extract was tested against six human cancer cell lines: lung, liver, cervical, breast, ovarian, and colon cancer. Amla not only stopped the cancer growth completely but also killed the existing cancer cells, reducing their population by over 50 percent, and significantly blocked the cancers' ability to spread.[10] Another study showed that just ¾ teaspoon per day of dried amla powder worked better at lowering high blood sugar into a normal range than the diabetes medication glyburide. In addition to regulating blood sugar, the study also found that the equivalent of one gooseberry per day cut bad cholesterol and triglycerides in half and boosted good cholesterol after only three weeks of supplementing daily.[11] Food trumps pharmaceuticals!

TIP:

Berries are one of the most pesticide-contaminated crops, which is why you should always buy them organic.

One small problem with amla, though, is that it tastes terrible. It is bitter, sour, pithy, and just plain awful. The first way I ever had amla was in an herbal fruit paste from India called Dabur Chyawanprash, which is a thick brown paste that's sweet and spicy.

But years later, when I first tried an amla berry whole . . . wow, was it gross. The easiest way to get amla in your body is by adding organic dried amla powder to water, juice, or a smoothie. You can get organic amla/amalaki powder online.

I'm often asked, "If sugar feeds cancer, what about the sugar in fruit?" The naturally occurring sugars in fruits and vegetables provide energy to every cell in your body, and the antioxidants and phytonutrients provide a wide range of anti-inflammatory and anti-cancer benefits in the body. Fruit is a wonderful health-promoting food, and nearly every fruit on earth has been found to contain anti-cancer compounds. I don't worry about the naturally occurring sugars in whole fruit. If there's one thing I'm sure of, I didn't get cancer from eating too much fruit.

THE TOP 10 ANTI-CANCER VEGETABLES

In January 2009 researchers published a study in the journal *Food Chemistry* comparing the anti-cancer effects of 34 vegetable extracts on eight different tumor cell lines. Researchers basically just ran vegetables through a juicer and then dripped the juice on different cancer cells to see what would happen. Many of the vegetables had significant anti-cancer effects, but the most powerful anti-cancer vegetable was garlic.

Garlic stopped cancer growth completely against the following tumor cell lines: breast cancer, brain cancer, lung cancer, pancreatic cancer, prostate cancer, childhood brain cancer, and stomach cancer. Leeks ran a close second and were number one against kidney cancer. But garlic and leeks weren't the only superstars: almost every vegetable from the allium and cruciferous families completely stopped growth in the various cancers tested. The allium family vegetables tested were garlic, leeks, yellow onions, and green onions. The cruciferous family veggies tested were broccoli, Brussels sprouts, cauliflower, kale, red cabbage, and curly cabbage. Spinach and beet root also scored in the top 10 against many of the cancers tested. Honorable mentions include asparagus, green beans, radishes, and rutabaga. Here is an excerpt from the study:

The extracts from cruciferous vegetables as well as those from vegetables of the genus *Allium* inhibited the proliferation of all tested cancer cell lines whereas extracts from vegetables most commonly consumed in Western countries were much less effective. The antiproliferative effect of vegetables was specific to cells of cancerous origin and was found to be largely independent of their antioxidant properties. These results thus indicate that vegetables have very different inhibitory activities towards cancer cells and that the inclusion of cruciferous and *Allium* vegetables in the diet is essential for effective dietary-based chemopreventive strategies.[12]

The most powerful anti-cancer veggies in this study, including dark leafy greens, cruciferous veggies, and garlic, account for less than 1 percent of our Western diet. Something else worth noting in this study is that radishes were shown to stop tumor growth by 95 to 100 percent for breast and stomach cancer but had no effect and may have even increased tumor growth in pancreatic, brain, lung, and kidney cancer.

Researchers at Cornell conducted a similar study in 2002 in which they dripped the extracts of 11 common vegetables on human liver cancer cells. Spinach showed the highest liver cancer stopping power, followed by cabbage, red pepper, onion, and broccoli.[13] Garlic and leeks were not included in their study. Most of the top anti-cancer vegetables identified in both studies are the same vegetables I ate twice per day every day in a giant salad. The only veggies I did not eat were leeks, radishes, and rutabaga because I had no idea they were so great.

Brocc-Out and Crucify Cancer Cells

High intake of cruciferous vegetables including broccoli and cauliflower has been associated with reduced risk of several cancers such as breast cancer and aggressive prostate cancer.[14,15] Here are a few clues as to why. Your immune system begins in your intestines, and your body's first line of defense against pathogens, bacteria, viruses, parasites, and cancer-causing toxins are immune cells called intraepithelial lymphocytes. These cells are covered in aryl hydrocarbon receptors. Broccoli and other cruciferous veggies contain an anti-cancer compound called indole-3-carbinol, which activates the aryl hydrocarbon receptors on your intraepithelial lymphocytes, supercharging your intestinal immune cells. Broccoli also contains a compound called sulforaphane, which is created by a chemical reaction that happens when you chop or chew raw broccoli and is the most potent phase 2 liver detoxification enzyme known. If you plan to cook cruciferous veggies, chop them 30 to 40 minutes before cooking to allow the sulforaphane reaction to take place.

Broccoli sprouts contain roughly 25 times more sulforaphane and 100 times more indole-3-carbinol than mature broccoli, and they can be found in the refrigerated produce section of most grocery stores right next to the alfalfa sprouts. You can also purchase broccoli seeds and sprout them in three to four days at home, which makes them the cheapest and most powerful immune-boosting and detoxifying medicinal food on earth. Broccoli sprouts should be eaten raw and are great on salads. I should note that it is possible to get too much of a good thing. Too much sulforaphane could be toxic and make you feel sick, so it's recommended that you do not eat more than four cups of broccoli sprouts per day. Two to three cups per day should keep you on the safe side.

Medicinal Mushrooms

Mushrooms are a powerful immune-boosting, health-promoting food, and daily intake of mushrooms may have significant anti-cancer properties for many cancers, including breast cancer. Estrogen-positive (ER+) breast cancers need estrogen to grow, but simply eliminating estrogen from the diet may not be enough because many breast cancer tumors can synthesize their own estrogen by converting testosterone to estrogen with an enzyme called aromatase.

In one study, white button mushrooms were shown to suppress aromatase by 60 percent, which was better than any other vegetable and mushroom tested.[16] Mushrooms also boost your immune system and reduce inflammation in your body. Eating one cup of cooked white button mushrooms per day is shown to accelerate the salivary secretion of an immune system antibody called immunoglobulin A by 50 percent.[17] That's a very good thing.

Some of the powerful anti-cancer compounds found in mushrooms, oats, barley, and nutritional yeast are polysaccharides called beta-glucans. They are known as "biological response modifiers" because of their ability to activate the immune system.[18] Simply put, they make your immune system work better. Beta-glucan supplementation has even been tested on endurance athletes like cyclists and marathon runners. It's not uncommon for endurance athletes to get sick after a long race because extreme exercise causes immune suppression, but in one study, a control group taking beta-glucans cut their post-race infection rate in half.[19]

The rate of breast cancer in American women is six times higher than in Asian women. Two protective dietary factors that have been identified are green tea and mushrooms. In 2009 researchers found that Chinese women who ate an average of only 15 mushrooms per month along with drinking 15 cups of green tea per month had an astounding 90 percent reduced risk of developing breast cancer when compared to Chinese women who didn't consume green tea or mushrooms regularly.[20]

Drinking green tea and eating mushrooms daily could have a significant impact on your health. I ate raw mushrooms daily in my giant salads, but recent studies indicate that it might be better to eat mushrooms cooked because cooking destroys a toxin found in raw mushrooms called agaritine. If you really don't like the taste of mushrooms or you just want to maximize your immune benefit from mushrooms, you can also take them as supplements from a reputable company like Host Defense or Mushroom Wisdom.

Turmeric

The turmeric plant is a relative of ginger and has been used for thousands of years in Indian ayurvedic medicine as an antiseptic and antibacterial agent to heal wounds and treat infection, inflammation, digestive issues, and more. Indians eat a mostly plant-based diet with some of highest spice consumption in the world, and have significantly lower cancer rates than Western countries.[21] Indians have roughly 9 times less melanoma, endometrial cancer, and kidney cancer, 5 times less breast cancer, 10 times less colorectal cancer, 7 times less lung cancer, and 23 times less prostate cancer.[22]

Turmeric is one of the most powerful cancer-fighting spices known because it contains the anti-inflammatory antioxidant polyphenol curcumin, which has been shown to inhibit growth of many types of cancer cells.

Curry powder, a spice mix commonly found in Indian, Middle Eastern, Thai, and Malaysian cuisine, typically includes turmeric, coriander, cumin, chili peppers, and fenugreek and may also include clove, cinnamon, cardamom, fennel, and ginger. I love turmeric and curry powder, and I put them on nearly everything I eat. I even put a teaspoon of turmeric in oatmeal and a tablespoon in fruit smoothies.

Most cancer drugs target only one cancer pathway. For example, 5-FU targets DNA and methotrexate targets folic acid reductase. Curcumin, the active anti-cancer compound in turmeric, targets at least 80 cancer-linked cell-signaling pathways like p53, tumor necrosis factor, interleukin-6, NF-kB and mTOR.[23] Curcumin has the ability to block every stage of cancer development, from cancer formation to tumor growth to metastasis. It can also kill many different types of cancer cells by triggering apoptosis (programmed cell death) without harming normal cells.

Multiple clinical studies have found that doses of 8 grams per day of curcumin had no toxic effects in humans.[24] One study on Curcumin C3 Complex reported no toxic effects in humans taking 12 grams per day.[25] To date, a maximum daily dose has not been identified. Curcumin reaches peak blood concentrations in one to two hours. Taking it three times per day keeps therapeutic levels fairly consistent. A number of studies have shown that high-dose curcumin supplementation (8 grams per day) can enhance the effectiveness of chemotherapy drugs.[26] But in some cases, high-dose curcumin could cause adverse effects, depending on which drugs it is combined with. *Exercise extreme caution.* Dr. Bharat Aggarwal, curcumin researcher and author of more than 600 scientific papers, recommends dosing gradually starting with 1 gram per day for the first week and doubling the daily dose each week. By week 4 you will be taking 8 grams per day. In 2017 the *British Medical Journal* published the first ever case report of a woman who reversed her late-stage myeloma by taking 8 grams of Curcumin C3 Complex with BioPerine per day.[27] BioPerine is a patented formulation of piperine, an extract of black pepper or long pepper, which has been found to increase the absorption of curcumin by 2000 percent.[28]

Oregano

Oregano is an antibacterial, anti-inflammatory, and anti-cancer spice with high levels of antioxidants and antimicrobial compounds. Oregano ranks as one of the top ten highest antioxidant spices on earth, and one teaspoon of oregano has the same antioxidant power (oxygen radical absorbance capacity, or ORAC) of two cups of red grapes. It contains the flavonoid quercetin, which is known to slow cancer growth and promote apoptosis. It is also a good source of vitamin K and iron. Laboratory studies have found oregano extracts to cause cancer cell death in colon cancer, breast cancer, and prostate cancer.[29, 30,31]

Garlic

Garlic is one of the most powerful anti-cancer vegetables. Numerous studies have shown it to lower the risk of developing all types of cancers, especially colon, stomach, intestinal, and prostate cancer. It has strong antibacterial properties as well as the ability to block formation and halt activation of cancer-causing substances. It can also enhance DNA repair, slow down cancer cell reproduction, and, like turmeric and oregano, induce apoptosis. The World Health Organization even recommends that adults eat one clove of fresh garlic per day.[32] I consumed several cloves per day during my most intensive cancer healing season. I often chopped the cloves up into tiny bits and downed them with a swig of water or juice.

Black garlic is a super potent form of garlic that involves aging garlic for 40 days in 140 to 170 degrees Fahrenheit with 85 to 95 percent humidity, which produces sweet, chewy cloves that are less pungent and easier to eat. As powerful as garlic is against cancer, black garlic has been found to have even higher antioxidant, anti-inflammatory, and anti-cancer activity.[33]

Cayenne Pepper

Cayenne pepper, like most hot peppers, contains capsaicin, the active compound that sets your lips, tongue, and everything else on fire. Capsaicin has been shown to alter the expression of several genes involved in cancer cell survival, growth, angiogenesis, and metastasis. Like curcumin in turmeric, capsaicin has been found to target multiple signaling pathways, oncogenes, and tumor-suppressor genes in various types of cancer models.[34] And the hotter the better. Cayenne will spice up your salad quickly, so go easy on it the first time. If you can handle the heat, habanero peppers contain four to six times more capsaicin than cayenne, with a Scoville rating of 200,000 units.

TEA UP

Another key component of an anti-cancer diet is drinking copious amounts of herbal teas, specifically the ones reported to have immune-boosting, detoxification, and anti-cancer properties. Here are a few of the teas known to be the least friendly to cancer.

Essiac Tea

This herbal tea made from burdock root, sheep sorrel, rhubarb root, and slippery elm bark was discovered by Canadian nurse Rene Caisse in 1922. (*Rene* is like Irene without the "I". *Essiac* is Caisse spelled backward.) As the story goes, Rene obtained the formula from a woman who had been given the formula by an Ojibwan Indian medicine man and used it to cure her own breast cancer 20 years prior. Two years later Caisse used the tea to cure her aunt of terminal stomach and liver cancer and her mother of liver cancer. Caisse opened a clinic and treated cancer patients with the herbal formula for 18 years until Canadian government pressure and litigation forced her to close it down. Despite numerous offers, Caisse was very protective of the formula and refused to sell it for profit.

In 1959 she partnered with Dr. Charles Brusch to continue research on the formula. Dr. Brusch expanded the formula adding watercress, blessed thistle, red clover, and kelp and used it to treat cancer patients in his clinic. He even used it to cure his own bowel cancer. In laboratory studies, Essiac tea has been shown to have five times the antioxidant power of green tea and has significant anti-cancer effects by inhibiting tumor growth and stimulating immune response for various cancers.[36] Two reputable brands are Essiac Tea made by Essiac Canada International and Flor-Essence made by Flora. Essiac tea only requires a small dose of 1 to 3 ounces, two to four times per day. You can also make your own, as the formula is now widely known. I recommend the Essiac tea instructional videos by Mali Klein on YouTube.

TIP:

Metal cookware and tea kettles can leach metals like nickel and chromium into your tea, including stainless steel.[35] Try using a ceramic or glass teakettle.

Jason Winters Tea

In 1977 Jason Winters was diagnosed with terminal cancer and given three months to live. With nothing to lose, he decided to travel the world in search of a cure. He discovered medicinal herbs used for centuries on three different continents to promote healing in the body: red clover, chaparral, and a Chinese herbal tonic known as Herbalene, which contains astragalus and *Ligustrum*. The individual herbal remedies had little effect when consumed separately, and his condition worsened. As a last-ditch effort, he combined them all together in a tea and proceeded to drink about a gallon per day, and the large tumor on his neck began to shrink and was gone in three weeks. After his recovery, he began selling this blend, now known as Jason Winters Tea. In the last 30 years, research has shown that the herbs in Jason Winters Tea appear to have blood purification and immune supporting properties.[37,38] Chaparral has anti-cancer activities.[39] Astragalus has antioxidant, anti-inflammatory, immunostimulant, anti-cancer, and anti-viral activities.[40] Red clover has antioxidant activity and is also an aromatase inhibitor.[41,42]

Jason Winters wrote a book documenting his experience called *Killing Cancer*. He dedicated the rest of his life to health education and won numerous awards around the world, including being knighted in Malta in 1985. Jason Winters Tea is delicious and naturally caffeine free. Our kids call it "Jason tea," and we love to drink it iced at our house.

Dandelion Root Tea

This pesky weed that pops up in your yard every spring is a powerful anti-cancer plant. Dandelion root tea has been shown to kill various types of cancer cells in the lab and in animals, including those for colon cancer, breast cancer, leukemia, melanoma, and even pancreatic cancer without harming healthy cells.[43,44,45,46,47]

Making dandelion root tea is simple. Dig up a dandelion that hasn't been sprayed with weed killer, cut off the root, and chop it or grind it up. Put ½ teaspoon to a teaspoon in a tea bag, steep it in boiling water for 20 minutes, and drink two or more cups per day. Dandelion root tea and dandelion root extract can be found at health food stores and ordered online. Don't throw away the dandelion greens. They are also highly nutritious and can be added to a salad or blended up in a smoothie. Don't eat the puffball.

Green Tea

The practice of drinking green tea dates back over 1,000 years to the Tang dynasty in China. Green tea contains known anti-cancer phytonutrients called catechins (epigallocatechin gallate, or EGCG) and about 13 times more antioxidants than blueberries and pomegranates. Regular consumption of green tea has been associated with a lower risk of death from cardiovascular disease and death from all causes.[48] It has also been shown to reduce the risk of certain cancers including breast cancer, prostate cancer, and colon cancer.[49] Matcha green tea is considered to be the most nutritious form of green tea. The matcha process involves grinding young green tea leaves into a fine powder that dissolves in water. (You don't have to grind it up; it comes that way.) And unlike steeping tea in a tea bag, you're consuming the entire tea leaf so you get all the nutrients. Green tea is wonderful and matcha green tea may be even better. You can drink matcha green tea hot or cold or add it to juice or smoothies.

Hibiscus Tea

Recent research has shown that hibiscus tea has an even higher antioxidant content than green tea. It is also rich in phenolic acids, flavonoids, and anthocyanins. Hibiscus extracts have been shown to inhibit the growth of cancer cells in the lab and have beneficial effects on inflammation, atherosclerosis, liver disease, diabetes, and other metabolic syndromes, which are all good reasons to drink it. Celestial Seasonings organic Zinger teas are all hibiscus-based teas.[50] You can also buy dried organic hibiscus in bulk, brew it yourself, or blend it into your smoothies, water, or juice.

FOOD FOUNDATIONS

Healing cancer does not require a secret formula, an exotic Amazonian plant, or a therapy costing tens of thousands of dollars. Cancer patients don't have to climb remote mountaintops to access a hidden cure. Nor do they have to fork over every dollar they have to access expensive treatments only available to a select few. Fruits, vegetables, mushrooms, spices, nuts, seeds, and herbal teas are the foundational ingredients of the anti-cancer diet. The truth is simple: whole foods from the earth give your body vital nutrients that enable it to repair, regenerate, detoxify, and heal.

Whether you have cancer or you want to prevent it, hopefully now you have a sense of how important your dietary choices are. The food on the end of your fork has the power to promote health or promote disease. Choose wisely.

HEROIC
DOSES

The Anti-Cancer Diet

If man made it, don't eat it.

— JACK LALANNE

IN THE OLD TESTAMENT OF THE BIBLE, the Book of Daniel records a period of time when the Jewish people were living as captives of their conquerors in Babylon. The Babylonian king Nebuchadnezzar ordered young men from the Israelites' royal family to be trained to serve in his palace for three years. Daniel was one of those men.

The king ordered that the young men be fed the food from his table, but Daniel, in order to not violate his religious tradition, asked the chief official for permission not to eat the king's food. The official refused. Daniel then said, "Please test your servants for ten days: Give us nothing but pulse to eat and water to drink.

Then compare our appearance to the rest of the men who eat the royal food, and see what happens."

The word "pulse" refers to plant food like whole grains, beans, peas, fruits, vegetables, nuts, and seeds—whatever was available in that region at the time. Daniel was given permission to do the test, and after just 10 days he and his friends who chose to eat humble plant food from the earth appeared remarkably healthier and more nourished than the young men who ate the king's finest fare. Was their improved health a miracle or was it the diet?

Twenty-seven hundred years later and two blocks from my house, researchers at the University of Memphis put 43 relatively healthy participants on a 21-day "Daniel fast," eating a strict plant-based (vegan) diet of fruits, vegetables, nuts, and seeds with no animal food as well as no processed food, additives, preservatives, white flour, sweeteners, caffeine, or alcohol. At the end of 21 days, the participants had significant increases in antioxidant capacity and nitric oxide in their blood—both very good things. They also had reductions in oxidative stress, blood pressure, cholesterol, insulin levels, insulin resistance, and C-reactive protein, a marker of inflammation in the body.[1] In just 21 days, eating a whole-food, plant-based diet significantly improved their risk factors for metabolic and cardiovascular disease. Just like Daniel and his mates, they got healthier. A king's diet is not a healthy diet. It is a diet of excess. The king's diet in Daniel's day sounds a lot like the diet most of us eat today—a diet rich in meats, cheeses, sweets, and alcohol.

THE ANTI-CANCER DIET IS A PLANT-BASED DIET

The first phase of my Massive Action Plan to heal cancer was essentially an amped up 90-day Daniel Fast. I was determined to live and to change my internal terrain in order to make my body an environment where cancer could not thrive. Step one in this process was eliminating all processed man-made food and animal products in favor of an organic, whole-foods, plant-based diet.

In 2005, medical doctor and clinical researcher Dean Ornish at the University of California San Francisco, along with colleagues from UCLA and Memorial Sloan Kettering Cancer Center, conducted a study which proved that the progression of early stage prostate cancer can be reversed with intensive diet and lifestyle changes, specifically a low-fat, whole-foods, plant-based diet, exercise, and stress reduction. The 44 patients in the study who adopted a plant-based diet and incorporated daily exercise and stress management techniques instead of conventional therapy had a 4 percent drop in their PSA cancer-marker counts on average after one year. A 4 percent drop may not sound like much, but it indicates that their cancer had stopped spreading and that their bodies were healing. The patients with the strictest compliance to the diet and lifestyle program had the best improvement.

Meanwhile, the 49 patients in the control group, who didn't make any diet and lifestyle changes, had an average 6 percent increase in their PSA counts after one year, indicating disease progression. Researchers took the blood of the patients put on a plant-based diet for one year, dripped it directly onto cancer cells, and found that it had eight times the cancer stopping power. The plant-based patient blood slowed down the growth of prostate cancer cells in the lab by 70 percent. The blood of the control group eating the standard American diet (SAD) only slowed cancer growth by 9 percent.[2]

Another study took ten men with advanced prostate cancer whose PSAs were rising after having their prostates removed and put them on a similar program, which included a low-fat, whole-foods, plant-based diet and stress management. After four months, five of the ten patients had significantly slower PSA growth and three of the patients had lower PSAs than when they started, indicating disease reversal. Only two patients did not show improvement.[3] Just as in the Ornish study, those who committed to the program and followed it as directed had the best results.

In 2006 some of the same researchers from the Ornish study conducted a similar study on breast cancer cells. They took blood from overweight and obese postmenopausal women eating a standard American diet and dripped it on three different types of breast cancer cells. The SAD blood had only a small effect in suppressing the growth of the breast cancer cells. Then they put the women on a low-fat, whole-foods, plant-based diet and had them take an exercise class every day. Twelve days later they took more blood samples from the same women and dripped their blood on the breast cancer cells again. After just 12 days on a whole-foods, plant-based diet with daily exercise, the women's blood stopped the cancer cell growth between 6 and 18 percent and increased apoptosis (programmed cell death) between 20 and 30 percent.[4]

In 2015 after reviewing 800 scientific studies, the World Health Organization's International Agency for Research on Cancer (IARC) classified processed meats including bacon, sausage, ham, corned beef, canned meat, and jerky as Group 1 carcinogens. That means these foods directly cause cancer. They reported that eating 50 grams or 1.75 ounces of processed meat per day—that's only about two strips of bacon—increases your risk of colorectal cancer by 18 percent.[5] The IARC also classified red meat as a Group 2A carcinogen, which means there is limited evidence indicating that it probably causes cancer. The highest risk is for colorectal cancer, but links between red meat and processed meat consumption and pancreatic cancer and prostate cancer were also reported. Another meta-analysis associated increased consumption of red meat and processed meat with colorectal, esophageal, liver, lung, and pancreatic cancers.[6]

Will eliminating processed meat and red meat from your diet cut your cancer risk? Absolutely. But that's just one part of the equation. Eating animal products can also promote the growth of cancers in a number of ways.

One significant anti-cancer effect of a whole-foods, plant-based diet appears to be its ability to reduce insulin-like growth factor-1 (IGF-1) in the body. IGF-1, a growth hormone directly linked to uncontrolled cancer growth, increases in your body when you eat a diet high in animal protein and/or refined sugar. After just two weeks on a whole-foods, plant-based diet, the blood of breast cancer patients was found to have significantly lower levels of IGF-1 and increased cancer stopping power.[7]

Many human cancer cells, including colorectal, breast, ovarian, melanoma, and even leukemia, are dependent on an amino acid called methionine.[8,9] Without it, they die. Methionine is one of nine essential amino acids that cannot be made by the body. It must come from food. And guess which food group has the highest levels of methionine: animal foods! One way to deprive cancer cells of methionine and control cancer growth is to stop eating animal foods. Overall, fruits contain little to no methionine. Vegetables, nuts, and whole grains have small amounts of methionine. The highest source of methionine in the plant kingdom is beans, but animal foods have more. Milk, eggs, and red meat have more than twice as much methionine as beans, and chicken and fish have five to seven times more.

Beans, split peas, chickpeas, and lentils contain a valuable anti-cancer compound called inositol hexaphosphate, also known as IP6 or phytic acid. IP6 has been found to reduce cell proliferation and contribute to tumor cell destruction. It's even been shown to enhance the anti-cancer effects of chemotherapy, control cancer metastases, and improve quality of life.[10]

A 2014 study found that middle-aged Americans ages 50 to 65 who reported eating a high-protein diet with more than 20 percent of calories coming from animal protein were four times more likely to die of cancer or diabetes and twice as likely to die of any other cause in the next 18 years. But those who ate a plant-based diet did not have any increase in risk.[11] A diet high in animal protein is typically also high in saturated fat. A diet high in saturated fat has been found to increase your risk of lung, colorectal, stomach, and esophageal cancer.[12,13,14] It also increases your risk of breast cancer if you're a woman and prostate cancer if you're a man.[15,16]

Another cancer promoter found in animal food is heme iron, a highly absorbable form of iron found in meat—especially red meat, organ meat, and shellfish—but not in plant food. In small amounts, iron is good for the body and necessary for the formation of healthy blood cells, but in excess iron causes oxidative stress and DNA damage and can catalyze endogenous formation of N-nitroso compounds, which are potent carcinogens. Excess dietary iron has been linked to an increased risk of esophageal and stomach cancer as well as colorectal cancer.[17,18] Excess iron that is not used in blood cell formation accumulates in your liver, heart, and pancreas and can contribute to iron overload because your body has no way of ridding itself of iron except by bleeding. In addition, research published in 2018 concluded that two common forms of iron used in iron supplements, ferric citrate and ferric EDTA, might be carcinogenic as they increase the formation of amphiregulin in colon cancer cells, a known cancer biomarker most often associated with long-term cancer with poor prognosis.[19] Another form of iron, ferrous sulphate did not have this effect. A little-known benefit of menstruation is that women naturally shed excess iron every month until menopause. A 2008 VA Hospital study found that intentional blood iron reduction every six months in patients with cardiovascular disease resulted in a 37 percent drop in their cancer incidence and that those who developed cancer had a much lower risk of death.[20]

Non-heme iron is abundant in plant foods, especially in legumes, sesame seeds, pumpkin seeds, spinach, Swiss chard, quinoa, and dried apricots.

When you stop eating animal products and replace them with whole plant foods from the earth, you stop eating animal-derived protein and saturated fat; reduce the levels of cancer promoters like growth hormone IGF-1, methionine, and heme iron in your body; and increase the levels of thousands of anti-cancer phytonutrients found only in plant food.

PLANT POWER

For many years, the Centers for Disease Control and the National Cancer Institute have recommended that we eat at least 5 servings of fruits and veggies per day to protect against cancer, but a 2017 study concluded that eating 10 servings is even better. Eating 10 servings of fruits and vegetables per day (800 grams) was associated with a 24 percent reduced risk of heart disease, a 33 percent reduced risk of stroke, a 28 percent reduced risk of cardiovascular disease, a 13 percent reduced risk of all cancers, and a 31 percent reduction in premature deaths![21,22] Fewer than one-third of Americans eat the recommended five servings of fruits and vegetables per day. In addition, the fruits and vegetables most commonly consumed by Americans have the smallest amount of cancer-fighting nutrients. Our modern diet, loaded with animal products and processed food and deficient in fruits and vegetables, is not only polluting our bodies, but is also depriving us of essential anti-cancer compounds.

My anti-cancer dietary strategy was to "overdose on nutrition." I wanted to saturate my body with the vital nutrients in fruits and vegetables in order to give it all the fuel and firepower it needed to repair, regenerate, and detoxify, and I went way beyond the recommended daily allowances. I went from eating a typical American diet that might include 1 to 2 servings of fruits and vegetables on a good day to eating between 15 and 20 servings *every single day.*

The first book I read about healing cancer with nutrition recommended taking the plant-based diet a step further and eating like Adam and Eve in the Garden of Eden—all raw and all organic. Like most of the world in January 2004, I had never heard of the raw-food diet, and I was fascinated by it. There were no raw-food social media superstars back then, and I didn't have anyone to follow other than a handful of fringe health and wellness authors. But something about it made sense. I was fascinated by the idea of only eating organic fruits and vegetables straight from the earth. I loved the simplicity and purity of the raw diet, and I was excited to see what effect it would have on my body.

My anti-cancer diet had two major objectives. First, eliminate all foods that might be a burden to my body and promote cancer growth, like processed food and animal food. Second, "overdose" on nutrient-dense foods from the earth. I wanted to saturate my body with vitamins, minerals, enzymes, antioxidants, and the thousands of phytonutrients and anti-cancer compounds found in plant food. You can't accomplish this by taking a handful of supplements. This approach required massive action and my Massive Action Plan consisted of three main elements, aka the Super Health Triad:

1. Juices
2. The Giant Cancer-Fighting Salad
3. The Anti-Cancer Fruit Smoothie

JUICING

In order to understand the value of juicing, you need to understand what happens when you eat. When you chew food, you are essentially juicing it in your mouth. You are breaking it down into liquid form and splitting open the cell walls. Your saliva contains enzymes that begin the digestive process and enable nutrients to be absorbed by your body. The food particles that cannot be broken down by your digestive system, such as fiber, pass through and head out the back door. Chewing separates the fruit and vegetable nutrients from the insoluble fiber. The better you chew before you swallow, the more nutrients you will absorb from your meal. Juicing is a great way to extract massive amounts of nutrients from fruits and vegetables without having to sit down and chew through 20 pounds of vegetables per day. Juicing releases approximately 90 percent of the nutrients in food, which is about three times better than you can do with your teeth.

Another key factor is absorption. If your digestive tract is inflamed and overrun with bad bacteria, you may only be absorbing a small amount of the nutrients in the food you eat. Fresh juice is alive, nutrient rich, and easy for your body to absorb and use. Breaking down and digesting whole foods require a lot of energy, which is why eating a big meal will often make you sleepy. Sick people usually have an energy problem. They need nutrients and energy from food, but the energy required to digest food robs energy from the healing processes in the body. As a result, many late-stage cancer patients have difficulty absorbing nutrients from food. But when you drink freshly extracted juice, the vitamins, minerals, enzymes, and phytonutrients are quickly absorbed into your bloodstream, where they are carried to all the cells in your body with almost no digestive energy required.

In the beginning, I drank 64 ounces per day of straight carrot juice, broken up into roughly eight 8-ounce servings throughout the day. Then, as I did some research, I began adding more ingredients to it. There are a thousand different combinations of veggie juice, but I kept it simple and typically either drank straight carrot juice or one of the following combinations.

MY BASIC JUICE FORMULA

(ONE SERVING)

> 5 small carrots
> 1 to 2 celery stalks
> ½ beet root (and a few beet greens)
> 1 knuckle gingerroot

MY ADVANCED JUICE FORMULA

(TWO SERVINGS)

> 5 small carrots
> 1 to 2 celery stalks
> ½ beet root (and a few beet greens)
> 1 knuckle-sized piece of gingerroot (or as much as you can stand)
> 1 to 2 knuckles turmeric root (or as much as you can stand)
> ¼ to ½ lemon or lime, unpeeled
> 1 whole green apple, unpeeled
> 1 clove garlic (or as much as you can stand)

NOTE: A knuckle is the length from your fingertip to your first knuckle.

Juice all the ingredients together and determine how many ounces of juice your juicer yields. Then multiply the ingredients to the get the desired amount of juice you want to make each day.

These additional ingredients may be added after the fact to amp up the nutritional value:

1 scoop greens powder

¼ to 1 teaspoon amla powder

¼ to 1 teaspoon moringa powder

¼ teaspoon matcha green tea powder

2 to 6 ounces aloe vera gel

CARROTS

Carrots are rich in cancer-fighting nutrients. Carrot juice has more naturally occurring vitamin A, alpha carotene, and beta carotene than anything else on earth. One 8-ounce cup of raw carrot juice has over 45,000 IU of vitamin A, which promotes liver detoxification and is healthy, unlike the isolated synthesized vitamin A found in most supplements. Carrots are rich in vitamin B-6 and also contain vitamins E and K; minerals including sodium, potassium, calcium, magnesium, and iron; flavonoids and carotenoids such as lycopene; and lutein. All of these nutrients work together to feed your cells, support your body's ability to inhibit the growth of many different cancers, and stimulate the activity of your immune system. Carotenoids and vitamin A have shown a strong ability to inhibit cancer induction, not only by viruses, but from chemicals and radiation as well. At least part of this effect is from these nutrients acting directly on your genes.[23] Another powerful anti-cancer compound in carrots is falcarinol, a fatty alcohol (which sounds terrible, but isn't), and is also found in *Panax* ginseng. Falcarinol has been demonstrated to have antibacterial, anti-fungal, anti-inflammatory, immune-boosting, and anti-cancer properties in laboratory studies, specifically against leukemia and colon cancer.[24]

BEETS

Beets are one of the highest antioxidant vegetables, and, like carrots, they are also rich in carotenoids, lycopene, and vitamin A, with strong anti-cancer and anti-mutagenic activity. Beets contain a potent anti-cancer phytonutrient called proanthocyanidin, which gives them their color. They contain betaine (a natural anti-inflammatory compound), vitamin C, folate, manganese, and potassium. Beets have also been shown to help lower high blood pressure and increase athletic endurance. Make sure to juice both the beetroot and the greens.

CELERY

Like carrots, celery contains the anti-cancer compound falcarinol, along with vitamins A, C, and K; minerals like potassium, calcium, and magnesium; and many other phytonutrients, including polysaccharides, antioxidants, phenolic acids, and flavonoids. Two noteworthy anti-cancer flavonoids in celery are apigenin and luteolin. In May 2013 researchers at Ohio State University demonstrated that apigenin could stop breast cancer cells from inhibiting their own death.[25] In other words, it made the cancer cells mortal again, like normal cells. Apigenin blocks aromatase, an enzyme in the body that helps promote the cancer growth hormone estrogen, and inhibits breast and prostate cancer cells.[26] Apigenin has even been found to make cancer cells more sensitive to chemotherapy by activating a tumor-suppressor gene called p53.[27] Luteolin helps protect cells from DNA damage, and both apigenin and luteolin have been shown to be anti-angiogenenic.[28,29] Another good source of luteolin is artichokes, while parsley and chamomile tea have high concentrations of apigenin.

GINGER

Ginger is a powerhouse root that contains antioxidant, anti-inflammatory, and anti-cancer compounds.[30,31] Multiple studies have shown that ginger can inhibit tumor cell growth, slow down metastasis, induce cancer cell death, protect healthy cells from radiotherapy damage, and enhance the effectiveness of chemotherapy.[32,33,34] Fresh gingerroot is spicy, and a small slice or knuckle goes a long way. Go easy on it the first time you add it to your juice.

JUICING TIPS

First and foremost, it's important to buy organic produce for your juice. In the United States, most commercial nonorganic produce contains traces of toxic pesticides, fungicides, and herbicides. Having said that, if you do not have access to or cannot afford organic produce, don't let that stop you. The benefits still outweigh the risks; just juice what you can get.

Don't get too hung up on the juice formula or ratio. The type of juicer you use will determine how much produce you'll need, and you'll figure it out in no time. There are a thousand possible juice combinations, so have fun experimenting. Vegetable juice is wonderful for you. Just get it in your body. You can also dilute the juice with purified water if the taste is too strong.

I didn't juice leafy green vegetables because they didn't produce as much juice as fruits and root vegetables, and I always felt like I was wasting them. In addition, some leafy greens, such as spinach and kale, contain high levels of oxalic acid, which can be problematic for some people. I prefer to eat leafy greens whole in a salad or blend them up in a smoothie.

I often supercharge my juice with an organic greens powder. There are many brands on the market today, and they typically have a variety of ingredients like barley grass, wheat grass, chlorella, and spirulina, along with lots of sprouts and veggies. Greens powders are rich in chlorophyll, trace minerals, antioxidants, and enzymes. Some brands also sell them in individual serving packets, which are great for travel and green juice on the go.

When juicing large batches, the best practice is to store the juice in the fridge in airtight glass mason jars or recycled glass bottles. Fill the bottles all the way to the top, leaving as little air as possible. This will slow down oxidation and help keep your juice fresh and potent throughout the day. I recommend drinking juice in the early morning, mid-morning, lunchtime, afternoon, dinnertime, and finish what's left before bed.

If you're serious about juicing large amounts of produce every day, you will need a good juicer. Cheap ones tend to jam up or don't produce much juice, and can frustrate you to the point where you won't juice at all. I bought a $300 Champion Juicer with a commercial motor in 2004, and it served me well for over a decade before I replaced any parts on it. Omega, Green Star, and Breville are also high-quality brands.

To get the maximum amount of juice out of your produce, you can use a Champion Juicer as a grinder and then press the juice out with a Welles or Peoples hydraulic juice press, which will yield about 50 percent more juice. This two-step process can produce as much as 2 ounces more juice per pound of carrots than the Rolls Royce of juicers, the $2,400 Norwalk, at only a third of the cost.

If money is tight, look for a used juicer on eBay or Craigslist, or ask your friends on social media. Chances are, someone you know has a juicer collecting dust that they will give to you for free or lend to you indefinitely. Don't let your circumstances stop you. Ask for help. The most important thing is that you get on the juice!

I'm often contacted by people who are concerned that carrot or beet juice contains too much sugar and "sugar feeds cancer." While it is true that cancer cells feed primarily on glucose, so does every other cell in your body. All fruits, vegetables, grains, and animal protein are converted to glucose to feed your cells. Carrots and beets contain anti-cancer nutrients that can turn off cancer genes, interfere with cancer cell reproduction, block metastasis, and cause cancer cell suicide. In my opinion, the positive benefits of the phytonutrients and anti-cancer compounds in carrots, beets, and fruit far outweigh any potential negative related to their sugar content. We aren't getting cancer from eating too much fruit, carrots, or beets. Carrot juice and beet juice are staples in the legendary anti-cancer nutritional protocols from Dr. Max Gerson and Dr. Rudolph Breuss, and I've known many cancer survivors whose healing protocols included lots of carrot and beet juice. I never worried about the sugar content in carrots and beets, and I don't think you should either.

What about fruit juice? Some of the literature I read back in 2004 claimed that even freshly juiced fruit juice had too much concentrated sugar for cancer patients, so I avoided fruit juice and only ate fruit whole or blended up in smoothies. Since then my attitude toward fresh fruit juice has changed. There are some powerful anti-cancer compounds in fruit juices, especially green apple and lemon juice. The Gerson Therapy for cancer includes one serving of fresh orange juice every morning and several 50/50 green apple and carrot juices throughout the day. If you are concerned about the sugar in fruit juice, you can eat apples and oranges whole instead, but definitely don't skip the lemon juice.

MY DAILY JUICE ROUTINE

Store-bought fruit and vegetable juices are not recommended because they are often not fresh and has been processed, pasteurized, and preserved. Fresh, organic juice is the best strategy. Some health experts recommend drinking fresh juice immediately in order to get the most nutritional value, but fresh juice has been found to retain its enzyme and nutritional content for several days. Back in 2004 I didn't have the luxury of making a fresh glass of juice eight times per day, so I had to devise a system that was simple and sustainable. My number one priority was getting large amounts of juice in my body every day. So first thing every morning, I made one big batch of juice to last me throughout the day. I started with 5 pounds of organic carrots, which yield approximately 40 ounces of juice, and then I added gingerroot, beet root, celery, and other ingredients to get me to 64 ounces, which I drank throughout the day. Ideally 64 ounces of juice should be consumed as eight 8-ounce servings, every hour or so. Many holistic cancer clinics have their patients drink between 1 and 3 quarts of juice per day. On the Gerson Therapy, cancer patients drink 13 juices per day, once every hour. Think of juice as medicinal food. Hourly dosing is the best way to maintain high levels of nutrients in your blood throughout the day.

OVERDOSING ON NUTRITION

I wanted to ensure that my body was getting all the nutrition it needed to repair, regenerate, and detoxify, and as a result I ended up drinking so much carrot juice that I turned orange. Overdosing on carotenoids temporarily turns your skin yellowish orange; it's common in babies when they eat too much carrot or sweet potato mush. This phenomenon is called carotenemia, but one nurse thought I was jaundiced, a symptom of a sick liver. The major difference between jaundice and carotenemia is that jaundice turns your eyes yellow. If your skin starts to turn yellow/orange, don't worry; it will eventually go away after you cut back on carrot juice. It's not uncommon for cancer patients who have turned orange from carrot juice to be warned by their doctor that too much vitamin A can be harmful and damaging to the liver. This opinion is based on studies using isolated vitamin A supplements, not carrot juice.

THE GIANT CANCER-FIGHTING SALAD

The second component in my anti-cancer diet was eating the biggest, baddest salad on the planet. The reason behind this salad was simple. I wanted to put as many anti-cancer vegetables into my body as possible every day. When I first started the raw-food diet, I bought several raw-food recipe books, but many of the recipes were complicated and time consuming and didn't contain the large variety of foods I wanted to be eating daily, so the giant salad ended up being my staple meal for lunch and dinner. I didn't mind eating the same thing every day because it was quick to prepare and delicious. Plus, I didn't have to put any time into planning my meals; I knew exactly what to buy at the grocery store every week and I ate everything I bought. No waste! There's really no secret formula, but I did follow some guidelines: No meat, cheese, or store-bought salad dressing. Use organic produce if you can get it and afford it to reduce your exposure to toxic chemical pesticides, herbicides, and fungicides.

THE GIANT CANCER-FIGHTING SALAD

Leafy greens: for example, kale, spinach, Swiss chard, watercress, arugula

Broccoli or broccoli sprouts

Cauliflower

Purple cabbage

Slice of red, yellow, or green onion

Leeks

Red, yellow, or green peppers (I know these are technically fruits)

½ or whole avocado (and so is this)

Sunflower seeds

Almonds or walnuts (unsalted, raw, or roasted)

Sprouted garbanzo beans

Sprouted black lentils

Sprouted mung beans

All vegetables are wonderful. Feel free to add any others you like. Availability and pricing will vary based on the season. Also, soaking and sprouting unlock enzymes and nutrition in nuts and seeds and may make them easier to digest, but it is not mandatory. Unsprouted nuts and seeds are wonderful healthy foods as well. Legumes should be soaked and sprouted if consumed raw. Otherwise, cook them.

Fun with Fermented Food

Health starts in the gut, and it's not uncommon for sick people to have digestive problems and unhealthy guts. The causes: eating a diet rich in meat, dairy, and processed food; eating conventionally grown produce sprayed with glyphosate; and taking antibiotics, all of which can either directly damage the gut or promote the abundance of inflammatory, disease-promoting bacteria. A critical part of the health restoration process is healing your gut and rebuilding your digestive tract. The first step is eating tons of plant food, which is rich in starch and fiber (these are prebiotics) and serves as food for probiotics, the good gut bacteria. The second step is eating a small amount of fermented foods daily, which contains live cultures of probiotic bacteria. Fermented foods help repopulate your intestinal flora with good bacteria, which displace bad bacteria and can improve your digestion and immune function. Pickled vegetables like sauerkraut, kimchi, and pickles, as well as apple cider vinegar, are my preferred fermented foods.

Traditional sauerkraut is made with only three ingredients: cabbage, water, and salt. Kimchi is a spicy Korean version of sauerkraut typically consisting of fermented cabbage, onions, garlic, and pepper. Recognized as one of the top five "World's Healthiest Foods" by *Health* magazine, kimchi has high concentrations of vitamin C and carotene in addition to vitamins A, B1, B2, calcium, iron, and beneficial bacteria.

As the old saying goes, "The dose determines the poison." Fermented foods may end up being unhealthy if you consume too much. Asian cultures with the highest intake of pickled vegetables also have the highest incidence of stomach cancer. A meta-analysis of observational studies conducted in Korea and Japan found that a high intake of pickled vegetables was associated with a 28 percent increased risk of gastric cancer. Kimchi accounts for approximately 20 percent of sodium intake in the Korean diet, and the high amounts of sodium used in pickled foods may be the real culprit.[35] Knowing what I know now, I still don't see any problem with adding a small amount (¼ cup) of either sauerkraut or kimchi to my salads every day. Look for organic sauerkraut, kimchi, and pickles in the refrigerated section of your local grocer or health food store. When comparing brands, look for the one with the lowest amount of sodium.

MY ANTI-CANCER SALAD DRESSING

Apple cider vinegar (I love Bragg)

Extra virgin olive oil and/or extra virgin flax oil
(I recommend Bragg and Barlean's)

Organic oregano

Organic garlic powder

Organic turmeric or curry powder

Organic cayenne pepper

Organic black pepper

Bragg organic sprinkle (a blend of 24 herbs and spices)

Nutritional yeast (I recommend Bragg, again!)

Lightly drizzle olive oil or flax seed oil and organic apple cider vinegar to taste. If you don't like the taste of apple cider vinegar, lemon juice is a great addition or substitute for ACV. Sprinkle on the spices to taste.

NOTE: Some people who switch to a raw-food diet may experience gas and indigestion. That's normal at first. If your body isn't used to eating lots of plant food, it may take a few days or weeks to adapt. Chewing your food really well, eating fermented foods daily, and taking a high-quality digestive enzyme with meals can help your body adjust. If digestion is difficult or painful, try the Giant Cancer-Fighting Salad blended up as a smoothie or blended and cooked as a soup.

Oleocanthal, a compound in olive oil, has been found to kill cancer cells in the lab in less than an hour.[36]

THE GREEN SMOOTHIE

Another way to get all of these anti-cancer veggies into your body is to put all (or most of) the ingredients of the giant salad into a blender with 1 to 2 cups of purified water, liquefy it, and drink it. This is especially good if you cannot eat solid food, want to consume it on the go, or want to give your jaws a break from all the chewing. Liquefying in a blender also increases the amount of absorbable nutrients. A liquefied salad is going to taste a bit unusual, kind of like a cold, bland vegetable soup. Not very appetizing sounding, I know, but keep in mind that this is medicinal food. You aren't drinking it for the taste. Even if you have to hold your nose, do it. Just get it in your body. Another option with this blended-up salad concoction is to warm it up on the stove. If you want to keep it raw, just warm it up to around 100 degrees, spice accordingly, and eat it like soup. If you have a hard time digesting raw food (such as having painful cramps or bloating), it can also be fully cooked and consumed warm or cooled.

APPLE CIDER VINEGAR

Apple cider vinegar (ACV) is a staple in my salad dressing. If you've never had it, it's exactly what it sounds like—vinegar made from apple juice. It tastes like vinegar, but with an apple-y twist, and it is celebrated in the natural health world for its many uses. ACV is a fermented food rich in probiotics, enzymes, potassium, and polyphenols, which are antimicrobial and antibacterial.[37] Apple cider vinegar contains acetic acid, which can help increase nutrient absorption in your body. Anecdotally, it has also been reported to assist in healing allergies, infections, candida, acid reflux, arthritis, and gout, and to support detoxification and immune function. Whether all these claims are true, I can't say. All I know for sure is that it is, at the very least, healthy, and I love it.

Bragg organic apple cider vinegar is the best of the best. It's raw and unfiltered, leaving all the vital nutrients and enzymes intact, unlike most vinegars, which are pasteurized, filtered, processed, and nutritionally dead. Paul Bragg was a lifelong health crusader and mentor to Jack LaLanne. He literally wrote the book on apple cider vinegar and numerous other books on diet, exercise, and fasting, and was a true pioneer in the world of health and wellness. My mom had many of his books in her library until I absconded with them. You can find Bragg ACV at most grocery and health food stores. I also recommend Bragg organic extra virgin olive oil.

NUTRITIONAL YEAST

Nutritional yeast contains a type of fiber called beta-glucan, an immunomodulatory compound that enhances your body's defenses against infections and cancer.[38] Beta-glucans have been shown to increase immune function, specifically monocyte and natural killer cell activity against cancer.[39] In one study, breast cancer patients who were given a small amount of beta-glucan daily—the equivalent of $\frac{1}{16}$ of a teaspoon of nutritional yeast— had a 50 percent increase in monocytes in their bloodstream after just two weeks.[40] Beta-glucan supplementation has also been found to accelerate wound healing after mastectomy.[41] There have been over 20 studies in Japan showing beta-glucans can enhance the effects of chemo and radiotherapy treatment and improve survival and quality of life.[42] Nutritional yeast has a mild cheesy, nutty flavor and can be added to oatmeal, smoothies, salads, and pretty much anything you eat. Bragg is my brand of choice, and I also take beta-glucans in supplement form.

YOU'RE GONNA NEED A BIGGER BOWL

When I first started making the Giant Cancer-Fighting Salad, I quickly realized that our little soup and side salad bowls were not going to cut it, so I bought some giant bowls that hold over 6 cups. That's 6 servings of vegetables in one meal. Remember: 10 servings per day of fruits and vegetables are considered ideal for cancer prevention; cancer healing may require more. I ate two giant salads per day and drank eight glasses of vegetable juice, plus a fruit smoothie. I was giving my body an abundance of nutrition with 15 to 20 servings of fruits and vegetables per day, every day. Like I said before, massive action produces massive results. And that, my friend, is what massive action looks like.

Note: The salad really doesn't have to be "giant." I made big ones because that's what it took to fill me up. Obviously, not everyone needs to eat as much as I did. Just make your salads big enough to satisfy your appetite and not leave you hungry an hour later.

MY ANTI-CANCER FRUIT SMOOTHIE

Berries are the most potent anti-cancer fruits, but it can be difficult to get organically grown berries, and they tend to be expensive and often get moldy within a few days. The most practical way to consume berries is to buy them frozen and blend them up in smoothies. I buy large bags of frozen organic berries at Costco, which are typically a mix of blueberries, blackberries, raspberries, strawberries, cherries, and sometimes even cranberries.

Depending on the size of the smoothie I want, I use:

1 to 4 cups of frozen organic berries

A handful of leafy greens like spinach or kale

A handful of almonds or walnuts, or both

1 banana or 3 to 5 pitted dates

I also like to add the juice and meat of a young Thai coconut. Fresh coconut is a delicious addition to the smoothie, but it tends to be expensive and it is difficult both to find and to open. And it is not essential.

Blend all ingredients in a blender with 1 cup of purified water. Add more water gradually if it's too thick. Note: If the smoothie is too thin, it may run through you.

If you want to amp your smoothies up even more, consider adding any of the following: 1 to 8 ounces Stockton aloe vera gel; 1 teaspoon to 1 tablespoon turmeric powder; 1 teaspoon amla powder; 1 teaspoon moringa powder; ½ to 1 teaspoon matcha green tea powder; pineapple; papaya; goji berries; acai berries; mangosteen; cauliflower . . . you get the idea. If it's a fruit or a vegetable, throw it in there.

If you need to gain weight, add more nuts and seeds, such as hemp hearts or pepitas.

GO NUTS

A 7-year study found that stage III colon cancer survivors who ate at least 2 ounces (57 grams) of tree nuts per week—roughly 48 almonds or walnuts (that's only about 7 per day)—were 42 percent less likely to have their cancer return and 57 percent less likely to die from their cancer than those who did not eat nuts.[43] This benefit applied only to those eating tree nuts (almonds, walnuts, Brazil nuts, pistachios, and cashews) but not peanuts. The study did not differentiate between raw or roasted nuts, so it's safe to assume that the study participants ate a variety of both. Roasting almonds doubles the antioxidant activity and phenolic compounds in almond skins.[44] However, nuts aren't just good for colon cancer. Eating a handful of nuts and seeds every day cuts your risk of several types of cancer (including breast cancer and pancreatic cancer), as well as cardiovascular disease, neurodegenerative disease, and diabetes.[45]

MY DAILY ANTI-CANCER ROUTINE

Here's what a typical day looked like for me while I was healing cancer, and even now. One of my intentions was to live as closely to nature as possible, to sleep in total darkness, and to let the sun wake me up naturally instead of being jarred awake by the radio or an alarm buzzer.

Once I'm up the first thing I do every morning is hydrate. I drink 20 ounces of purified water and/or tea cold-steeped overnight and take supplements that should be taken first thing in the morning. An additional benefit of drinking several cups of water first thing in the morning is that it gets your bowels moving. Next is 10 to 20 minutes of aerobic exercise such as jogging, cycling, or rebounding (jumping on a mini-trampoline) to wake me up, get my heart pumping and my blood circulating, and get me sweaty. Aerobic exercise not only has anti-cancer benefits in the body, but it also makes you feel good and promotes detoxification via sweating. Afterward I take a quick shower and spend a few minutes to get my mind on track for the day by reading a devotional passage, praying and/or meditating, journaling, and making or reviewing my to-do list. Next I make all my juice for the day, roughly 64 ounces. This process takes the better part of an hour. I recommend making it fun. Play some music you love or listen to a podcast while you're running the juicer.

In the first 90 days of my healing journey, I skipped breakfast and drank juice throughout the morning until lunch; some days I snacked mid-morning on fruit such as a grapefruit or a green apple. If you need to gain or maintain weight, oatmeal or the fruit smoothie is a great breakfast option. Lunch and dinner every day was the Giant Cancer-Fighting Salad. Some days I snacked on nuts or fruit mid-afternoon. Most days before lunch and dinner, I bounced on the rebounder for 10 minutes to incorporate more exercise into my day and get my lymphatic system moving. When the weather was nice, we often walked the dog after dinner. After dinner and before bed, I finished any remaining juice, sometimes drank herbal tea, and tried to get into bed within a few hours after sundown.

BUILDING
A NEW BODY

Tell me what you eat, and I will tell you what you are.

— JEAN ANTHELME BRILLAT-SAVARIN

YOUR BODY IS MADE UP OF TRILLIONS OF CELLS, almost all of which are dying and being replaced continually throughout your life. Your intestines are regenerated every two to three days, your taste buds take ten days, your skin and lungs take two to four weeks, your red blood cells take four months, your nails take six to ten months, and your bones take about ten years. About every hundred days, most of your soft tissue has been replaced. Your body is a perpetual construction site. And your body is built with the food you eat. That's it. You built your body. You are what you ate.

The ability of the human body to adapt to and use so many different types of fuel to repair, regenerate, and sustain life is an amazing testament to the intelligent design of our Creator. No matter what we put in it, it manages to keep working, which is why it's so easy for us take our bodies and health for granted. But you can only do that for so long, because if your nutritional requirements are consistently not met, and you replace vital, life-sustaining food from the earth with artificial, man-made factory food and high amounts of animal products, your health will decline. It's only a matter of time. Healthy cells and tissues are replaced with weaker ones as they regenerate, nutrient reserves are depleted, and the body becomes vulnerable to disease. Progressively, after many years, critical systems begin to break down, like your cardiovascular system, your central nervous system, your endocrine system, your digestive system, your reproductive system, or your immune system. All of these systems are connected, and when one system becomes dysfunctional it affects the others. And that's about the time when you begin to develop chronic pain, acid reflux, high blood pressure, irritable bowel syndrome, and high blood sugar, warning signs of diseases such as diabetes, heart disease, or cancer.

It takes multiple generations of cell degradation to produce a sick body but, thankfully, not nearly as many to heal it. When you stop polluting your body and give it the highest-quality raw materials (whole foods from the earth), it will reward you by rebuilding a healthier body. This is why many people experience a significant, even dramatic improvement in health in as little as three months after a radical diet and lifestyle change.

As encouraging as that is, I must emphasize that restoring health is not a quick fix. The experience of many practitioners and patients who have healed cancer shows that it can take several years to fully heal, and from there you must maintain a healthy diet and lifestyle for life. Every time you sit down to eat, remind yourself that you are building a new body. Before that first bite, ask yourself, *Is this food going to promote health or disease in my body?* In this chapter, I will highlight some time-tested, scientifically validated dietary principles for maintaining lifelong health.

In January 2004 I began working with a clinical nutritionist who took a holistic approach. Instead of treating symptoms, his focus was on supporting my body's ability to heal itself by identifying and correcting functional deficiencies and toxicities such as heavy metals. Along with blood work, he had me send samples of my urine, saliva, hair, and stool to various labs across the country for evaluation. When all of these tests came back, we had a detailed picture of what was happening in my body. From there he recommended individualized nutraceutical and herbal supplements to support various functions in my body.

After 90 days on a raw diet, he suggested I add some cooked food. At that point I had accepted that I would be on a raw diet indefinitely, maybe for the rest of my life, but at the same time I was open to doing whatever it took to get well. My nutritionist was the only person besides my parents who believed I was doing the right thing, so I trusted his advice.

When you are sick, there's no place for dietary dogmatism. It is easy to become convinced that one diet is the best diet for everyone, especially if you initially have good results with it yourself, but it's important that you stay open to refining your approach in order to give your body the optimal diet that it needs to thrive. The raw diet can be a powerful detoxification and healing diet in the short term, but it may not be sustainable for some people long term, depending on body type and metabolism. I'm an ectomorph (skinny frame) with a high metabolism. At that point, I was super skinny at six-feet-two, 130 pounds, and although I was eating tons of food and felt good on a raw diet, I was having trouble gaining weight and looked like Jack Skellington from *The Nightmare Before Christmas.*

I was clinically underweight, and it was clear that I needed more calories than juicing and giant salads could provide, so I started eating some cooked vegetables at night along with my giant salad. Contrary to what I'd been led to believe by raw foodists, cooking does not destroy the nutritional value of food; it actually breaks down cell walls and makes certain nutrients in food easier to absorb. Cooking can reduce the amount of water-soluble vitamins by about 15 percent, but it also reduces the volume of the food so you end up eating more of it, so there's no net loss. If you've ever cooked spinach, you've seen how drastically the volume is reduced after cooking—a giant bag cooks down to a bowlful. This is why cooked vegetables are considered to have about twice the calories as raw vegetables.

After the first 90 days, I modified my diet from 100 percent raw vegan to about 80 percent raw and not vegan. At the recommendation of my nutritionist, I added some starches, including sweet potatoes, lentils, brown rice, and quinoa, and a few servings of clean animal protein per week. He suggested wild-caught Alaskan salmon or organic lamb. I had no desire to eat cooked food or meat at the time, but this modification did help me get back to my normal weight in a few months.

Over the years, I have experimented with increasing the amount of animal food in my diet, including eating more servings of wild-caught fish or organically-raised chicken, beef, eggs, and even raw dairy to see how these foods affected my body. But I found no additional benefit. In hindsight, adding a few servings of animal protein per week back to my diet clearly wasn't enough to hurt me, but if I knew then what I know now, like how elevated levels of IGF-1, methionine, saturated fat, and heme iron from eating animal protein can promote cancer growth, I would not have added it back to my diet so soon. I think the safest approach is to stay off all animal products for the first phase of your healing journey, at least 90 days and maybe for several years. Cancer doesn't develop overnight and doesn't heal overnight. Healing can take several years, with ups and downs along the way. It's important to be in it for the long haul, committed to the process and to a total life change, which is what is often required for healing.

THE CANCER PATIENT WHO FORGOT TO DIE

Diagnosed with terminal lung cancer in 1976, 66-year-old Stamatis Moraitis left the U.S. and moved back to Ikaria, a Greek island, to be close to his family and enjoy his last nine months on earth. He planted a garden and a vineyard, got lots of fresh air and sunshine, ate homegrown local food, slept late, took naps, ate and drank with friends at night, and started going to church. This was a radical change compared to his former life back in the United States, and as a result something unexpected happened. Or rather, something expected didn't happen. He didn't die. Thirty years later, he celebrated his 96th birthday a cancer-free man without any help from doctors or drugs. Not even any alternative therapies or juicing. Stamatis slowed down, simplified his life, adopted a whole-foods diet, and reconnected with God, old friends, and family, and his body healed.

Stamatis Moraitis is not an anomaly. The island of Ikaria is classified as one of five Blue Zones documented by National Geographic fellow Dan Buettner. The Blue Zones are unique areas around the world where the healthiest, longest-living people live. Ikarians live on average 8 to 10 years longer than Americans and are four times as likely to reach age 90 in better health with less depression and dementia. Here's what makes life on Ikaria unique: The pace of life is slow. People wake up naturally. No alarm clocks. No stressful morning rush. They eat fresh local food that they produce themselves. They get exercise working in their gardens and walking up and down the hilly terrain. They eat lots of plant foods like garlic, potatoes, and wild greens and six times as many beans per day than Americans, including garbanzo beans, black-eyed peas, and lentils. They also eat breads from stone-ground whole wheat.

Ikarians are not vegetarians or vegans, but they eat a lot less meat than we do, only about three to four times per week. Typically, it's fresh-caught fish about twice a week and other meats about five times a month. They drink fresh goat's milk and eat honey. They drink lots of herbal teas with wild marjoram, sage, mint, rosemary, artemisia, and dandelion. They eat very little processed food and consume 75 percent less refined sugar than Americans. They spend a lot of time socializing and sharing meals with each other, and often stay up late drinking and dancing. Sounds pretty nice, right?

Speaking of drinking, they drink on average two to three cups of coffee and two to four glasses of wine per day. Multiple servings of coffee and wine per day are not a good strategy for anyone trying to transform their health, but it appears that the overwhelming healthiness of the Ikarian diet and lifestyle counteracts any negative effects of those indulgences. It is also worth noting that Ikaria is not a rich place. In fact, it's the opposite. Unemployment is around 40 percent, but almost everyone has access to a family garden and livestock, and they share what they have with each other. *The Blue Zones: Lessons for Living Longer from the People Who've Lived the Longest* by Dan Buettner is one of my favorite books on health and longevity. I've interviewed Dan on my blog as well.

LESSONS FROM RURAL AFRICANS

Dr. Denis Burkitt was a world-renowned Irish surgeon and devout Christian who spent many decades working as a medical missionary in Africa. Burkitt has been immortalized in Cancerdom for his 1958 discovery of Burkitt's lymphoma, a children's cancer caused by the Epstein-Barr virus, but what he did after that made him a legend in epidemiology. After many years spent working in African hospitals, Burkitt became discontent with simply treating the effects of chronic Western diseases and more interested in identifying the causes in order to prevent them. He surveyed hundreds of doctors at hospitals across Africa and discovered that many chronic diseases common to industrialized nations simply didn't exist in rural Africa. Rural Africans weren't getting our most common cancers, heart disease, diabetes, Crohn's disease, hemorrhoids, hernias, ulcers, gall stones, appendicitis, or autoimmune diseases. And if they made it through the infectious disease gauntlet of childhood, they were likely to live to be over 100 and simply die of old age.

One of Burkitt's first conclusions was that the absence of chronic Western diseases in rural Africa had nothing to do with genetics. Black Africans living in major cities eating the same diet as white Africans suffered from the same chronic diseases as they did. When Burkitt investigated the diets of rural Africans, he noted that they ate a high-fiber, plant-based diet that consisted of starchy vegetables such as potatoes, yams, cassava, peas, and beans; whole grains such as corn, millet, sorghum, teff, and wheat; and fruits like bananas and plantains, when available and in season. Unlike the Western diet, there was very little white flour and white sugar and very little meat and dairy. Rural Africans were eating a naturally high-carbohydrate, high-fiber, low-fat diet. The chief reason behind this diet was poverty and availability. There weren't any supermarkets in the African bush. The food they ate was the food they grew. Meat was scarce, a luxury eaten only on rare and special occasions. Burkitt also found that in any region where a Western diet rich in meat, dairy, and refined foods was adopted, chronic disease rates skyrocketed within a few decades.

Now let's talk about poop. One aspect of Burkitt's research involved measuring the stool size and bowel transit times of people all over the world, and his findings were revelatory. According to Burkitt, rural Africans were a model of healthy bowel function in comparison to American and British people, but in order to understand why, we must first discuss the liver.

The liver is responsible for as many as 500 functions in the body, one of which is detoxification. Along with the kidneys, it filters your blood, collecting, processing, and eliminating toxins and metabolic waste products from your body. One of the ways it does this is by excreting bile, your body's toxic waste, into your intestinal tract to be carried out by your stool. The longer that food and liver bile remain in the bowel, the more potential they have to putrefy and release toxic by-products and create fecal mutagens that cause irritation, inflammation, and ulceration in your intestinal walls, leading to bowel diseases like diverticulitis, colitis, Crohn's disease, and colorectal cancer. Some of the toxins in your poop can be reabsorbed into your bloodstream, causing a vicious cycle of autointoxication—poisoning and polluting your body and creating perpetual work for your liver. Meat, dairy, and eggs contain no fiber; move through your digestive tract very slowly, causing constipation; and putrefy in your colon, leading to the problems described above. Starch and fiber from plant food move through your digestive system quickly, absorbing toxic liver bile and carrying it out before it can cause any harm.

In his research Burkitt noted that rural Africans typically pooped twice per day and when they did, a lot more came out.

They expelled four times more poop per day by weight than Americans, Europeans, and Australians. Compared to the small, hard, dark poops of Western diet eaters, the Africans' poop was much larger, softer, and lighter in color, with no straining required. And the Africans' average bowel transit time—the time it takes a meal to go from mouth to anus—was about a day and a half, while Western diet eaters typically took three to five days. Perhaps most alarming was Burkitt's discovery that elderly Western diet eaters could take two weeks or more to pass a meal.

To measure your bowel transit time, eat beets with a meal and then track the number of hours before you have beet-red poop.

Burkitt was adamant that the number of doctors, medical technology, and health care available had very little bearing on the overall health of a nation. And he was right. The U.S. has the highest health spending of any industrialized nation in the world per capita and some of the shortest life spans. We spend twice as much as the Japanese on health care, and they live three and a half years longer on average. Burkitt also famously stated that the overall health of a nation could easily be measured by evaluating its people's stools. By 1973 Burkitt had written 28 medical journal articles on the connection between nutrition and disease, and he believed a high-fiber diet was the key to health and Western disease prevention.

Burkitt's work is monumental but he made one mistake: reductionism—trying to pinpoint Western disease on a singular dietary factor, namely fiber. His work was largely responsible for the dietary fiber craze of the '70s and '80s that prompted food manufacturers to produce and promote "high-fiber" breakfast cereals like All-Bran and supplements like Metamucil, convincing the public that simply adding more fiber to our diets would make us healthier. At the time of Burkitt's research, rural Africans consumed four to six times more fiber per day than Western diet eaters, but we now know that the high amount of fiber wasn't the reason they avoided chronic Western diseases. Several decades after Burkitt's work was published, researchers reexamined the native African diet. They found that today it consists primarily of highly processed corn grits and provides only half the U.S. recommended daily allowance of fiber, but surprisingly, the rates of colorectal cancer in Africa were still 50 times lower than the United States. The researchers concluded that the low rate of colorectal cancer among Africans could not be due to "protective" dietary factors like vitamins, minerals, and fiber because the modern African diet was actually found to be deficient in many of those nutrients. They credited the extraordinarily low rates of colon cancer to an absence of "aggressive" dietary factors—namely, excess animal protein and fat—and to beneficial by-products produced by Africans' colon bacteria, which are also influenced by diet.[1] Less meat equals more health.

CLEAN MEAT

After my nutritionist recommended I add some clean (organic pasture-raised or wild-caught) animal protein back into my diet, I was inspired to revisit the dietary laws that God gave to the Israelites, which are detailed in the Book of Leviticus of the Bible. These were laws pertaining to which animals they were allowed to eat and which animals were "unclean" and forbidden to eat. I've read these dietary laws many times in my life, and I never really understood them. But after closer examination and research, I discovered why God put these laws in place.

God told the Israelites they could only eat land animals with split hooves that chew their cud, which includes cows, goats, sheep, and deer but excludes dogs, cats, rodents, rabbits, pigs, horses, and snakes. They were also allowed to eat any water animal with fins and scales, which includes most fish but excludes reptiles, shellfish, dolphins, seals, and whales. Birds including chicken, turkey, duck, and pheasant were allowed, but birds of prey and scavengers such as eagles, ravens, hawks, and vultures were not allowed. There's a common thread here. The land animals and birds they were allowed to eat were mainly herbivores that ate plants and insects but didn't kill and eat other animals.

God, in His infinite wisdom, forbade the Israelites from eating most carnivorous predatory animals and scavengers. The Israelites were also not allowed to eat or drink blood from *any* animal. What we know now, thanks to science, is that these guidelines actually make a lot of sense. Carnivorous animal flesh and all animal blood can contain high amounts of viruses, bacteria, parasites, pathogens, and heme iron. Making these foods off-limits was much simpler than trying to teach the complexities of biology and anatomy.

SCAVENGERS

Scavengers are animals that eat the remains of other dead animals and include birds of prey like vultures, as well as swine and shellfish. Even though they are smart and can make great pets, pigs are nature's garbage collectors, and they will eat anything, including decaying dead animals and their own poop. Pigs don't sweat, and they store the majority of toxins they collect in their fat. Barbecue is especially bad because of the carcinogenic compounds created in the smoking process.

Shellfish also clean up their environment. They absorb the toxins and pollution in our rivers, lakes, and oceans. Polonium, a by-product of uranium, has polluted the world's oceans as a result of nuclear weapons testing, sunken nuclear subs, satellites, isotope batteries, and waste dumping from nuclear power plants.[2] The majority of our exposure to radioactive polonium comes from eating fish and shellfish because radioactive waste bioaccumulates in fish tissue. The higher up the food chain a fish is, the more toxic it becomes. Researchers found that just one meal of mussels caused a 300 percent spike in polonium levels in human semen.[3]

A catastrophic amount of radioactive fallout from the Fukushima meltdown in Japan ended up in the Pacific Ocean. Within several days of the meltdown, low levels of radioactive iodine and cesium were detected in rain and drinking water, as well as in grass and milk samples all across the United States. Milk samples in San Francisco were found to have 10 times the legal limit of radioactive iodine, and the highest levels of radioactive iodine in rainwater were found in Boise, Idaho. Tokyo Electric Power Company admitted in August 2013 that around 300 tons of highly radioactive water had leaked out of storage tanks, but some research scientists believe it may have been a lot more. Researchers at Stanford reported that Pacific bluefin tuna are transporting radioactive waste from Fukushima across the entire North Pacific Ocean as they migrate from Japan to California.[4] Testing revealed that Pacific tuna meat contained 10 times more radioactive nuclides after Fukushima, along with already high levels of mercury. Other scavengers to avoid are catfish, crawfish, shrimp, crab, lobster, mussels, squid, and octopus.

The Israelites had specific dietary laws as to which animals they could eat and how the meat should be prepared. Meat prepared according to these ancient laws is called kosher. In order to be considered kosher, the animal must be free from disease or injury and slaughtered in a way that, if done properly, is instantaneous and painless. After all the blood is drained out and the internal fat is removed, the meat is soaked in clean water for 30 minutes and drips dry. Afterward, it is salted for about an hour to draw out more blood. Then it's washed three times in cold, clean water to remove the salt. Then it is dried, cut up, and packaged.

The cleanest, healthiest, most humane meat you can eat is either wild caught or killed and prepared in a kosher manner or organic pasture-raised kosher meat. If you do include a small amount of animal protein in your diet, this is the best way to limit your exposure to potentially harmful toxins and heme iron in meat.

PATHOGENS, VIRUSES, AND BACTERIA, OH MY!

What's grosser than gross? In 2013 *Consumer Reports* found fecal bacteria in over half of the packaged raw ground turkey meat and patties they tested. Some samples harbored other germs, including salmonella and *Staphylococcus aureus*. Ninety percent of the samples had one or more of the five harmful bacteria they tested for. Sixty percent of the samples had *E. coli*. Surprisingly, the organic ground turkey was just as contaminated with bacteria as the conventional varieties. And almost all the disease-causing organisms they found were antibiotic resistant, except for those found in organically raised or antibiotic-free turkey.[5]

But it's not just turkey. The Retail Meat Report published by the FDA in February 2013 found that 81 percent of turkey, 69 percent of pork chops, 55 percent of raw ground beef, and 39 percent of chicken parts in supermarkets were infected with an antibiotic-resistant superbug called *Enterococcus*, a bacteria that is also the third leading cause of hospital infections. The FDA report also found that 74 percent of poultry contained antibiotic-resistant salmonella.[6]

In recent years there has been a growing concern about the increase in antibiotic-resistant bacterial infections in humans. This problem is largely caused by the rampant overuse of antibiotics in the meat and poultry industry. They are overdosing livestock with antibiotics to keep them from getting sick while living in the unsanitary conditions of factory farms. Nearly 80 percent of the antibiotics sold are used on food-producing animals. Roughly 30 million pounds of antibiotics are used on animals every year, which is four times more than the amount of antibiotics used on humans.[7] The simple and obvious way to protect yourself from unnecessary antibiotic exposure is to stop buying and eating factory-farmed meat.

As far as bacterial content goes, ground meat is the worst. Hamburger meat can contain as much as 100 million bacteria per quarter-pound patty. This is why it is strongly recommended that burgers be cooked well done. But even if the meat is completely cooked, the dead bacteria still release endotoxins into your blood-stream and cause an immediate inflammation response through-out the body, which causes stiffening of your arterial walls and lung inflammation.[8,9] This reaction typically lasts about five to six hours, and eating animal products three times per day keeps the body in a state of endotoxemia, or chronic, low-grade inflam-mation that can eventually lead to a host of diseases, including Crohn's disease, heart disease, diabetes, and cancer.

COOKED MEAT IS SAFER . . . AND MORE DANGEROUS

As if all those bacterial endotoxins weren't bad enough, cooking meat releases mutagenic compounds called heterocyclic amines (HCAs) and polycyclic aromatic hydrocarbons (PAHs). These are cancer-causing chemicals formed when muscle meat such as beef, pork, fish, or chicken is cooked at high temperatures, as in barbecuing, baking, pan frying, or grilling over an open flame. HCAs and PAHs are linked to various cancers, including kidney, colorectal, lung, prostate, and pancreatic cancer.[10,11,12,13,14] One large study found that the people with the highest consumption of meat cooked at high temperatures had a 70 percent greater risk of developing pancreatic cancer compared with those with the lowest consumption of well-done meats.[15] Fried bacon and fried fish have the highest concentrations of these mutagens, about five times more than beef and chicken. Chicken cooked without the skin has been found to have twice the levels of mutagens as chicken cooked with the skin on.

Meat cooked medium-rare has two-thirds less cancer-causing compounds than meat cooked well done,[16] but when you eat undercooked meat you risk the exposure to live bacteria like salmonella and *E. coli*. Boiling meat, as in stews and soups, is the safest cooking method because it kills bacteria without causing carcinogens. In recent years, there have been some fascinating discoveries in the world of nutrition science with regard to safely cooking meat.

HERBS AND SPICES TO THE RESCUE

In multiple studies, researchers have found that marinating meat with various herbs and spices before cooking blocks the formation of heterocyclic amines and polycyclic aromatic hydrocarbons. One study found that a marinade blend containing garlic, ginger, thyme, rosemary, and chili pepper reduced HCA production by 90 percent in pan-fried beef.[17] Another study comparing different marinades on grilled beef steaks found that a Southwest marinade with paprika, red pepper, oregano, thyme, black pepper, garlic, and onion reduced HCAs by 57 percent. An herbal marinade with oregano, basil, garlic, onion, jalapeño, parsley, and red pepper reduced HCAs by 72 percent. A Caribbean marinade containing thyme, red pepper, black pepper, allspice, rosemary, and chives reduced HCAs by 88 percent.[18] A third study in *Food Control* found that a simple lemon juice marinade could reduce the PAH content by as much as 70 percent.[19] Thus, always marinate your meat before cooking.

FIGHT FREE RADICALS WITH HERBS AND SPICES

Free radicals are caused by oxidative stress from external factors like radiation or pollutants and are also the toxic by-products of normal cell metabolism, kind of like your car exhaust. Free radicals damage cells, proteins, and DNA and are associated with causing disease including cancer, Alzheimer's, and Parkinson's disease. Your body is constantly neutralizing free radicals with the antioxidants that it makes, such as glutathione and super oxide dismutase, and with the antioxidants you eat. The more antioxidants you can get from food each day, the better. Plant food is rich in antioxidants, but herbs and spices have some of the highest concentrations of all, and are an easy way to supercharge the health benefits of any meal. The "Magnificent Seven" spices with the highest antioxidant content are cloves, peppermint, lemon balm, allspice, marjoram, cinnamon, and oregano.

Sweet Potato Tips and Tricks

➤ Sprinkle a little cinnamon and allspice on a sweet potato for more antioxidant power than nearly a week's worth of Western-diet meals.

➤ Sweet potatoes are delicious raw—just slice them up and dip them in some hummus.

➤ Raw sweet potatoes have higher antioxidant content than cooked, and boiled sweet potatoes have more than baked.

➤ Always eat the potato skin. It has about 10 times more antioxidant content than starch.

DOES MEAT CAUSE CANCER?

One of the largest prospective studies on diet and cancer found that the incidence of all cancers combined is lower among vegetarians than among meat eaters.[20] Processed meats like bacon, sausage, ham, and hot dogs are classified as Group 1 human carcinogens, which means there is strong evidence that processed meats cause cancer, specifically colorectal cancer. Red meat, including beef, lamb, and pork, is classified as a "probable" cause of cancer and has been linked to prostate and pancreatic cancer. There are many studies associating the consumption of animal protein and fat with an increased risk of certain cancers.

But haven't humans been eating meat for thousands of years? Yes, but our dietary habits and food systems are very different from those of our ancestors. Americans are eating twice as much meat as our great-grandparents, and even they were eating more meat than many of the populations with the lowest cancer rates today. In addition, the processed and factory-farmed meat we are eating contains higher levels of fat, growth hormones, and contaminants. Considering the fact that half of men and one-third of American women are predicted to get cancer in their lifetime, it makes sense to imitate the diets of the people with the lowest cancer rates and to reduce our exposure to as many cancer-promoters as possible.

Our bodies are bombarded with toxins every day from three sources: our environment, our food, and the products we use. We have limited control over our exposure to environmental toxins, many of which are undetectable, but we have complete control over what we put in and on our bodies. The goal is to reduce your toxic load. I believe giving up all animal products is essential for anyone who is trying to reverse a chronic disease like cancer.

Even if you don't have cancer, cutting out processed foods and eating less meat and more plant food can have a significant impact on your health in both the short and long term. Financial guru Dave Ramsey is famous for saying, "Live like no one else now, so later you can *live* like no one else." The same wisdom applies to your health. If you live and eat the way everyone else does, you can expect to get the same chronic diseases everyone is getting.

It is human nature to look for the quick fix, the one thing we can consume to be healthy, but there is no single cause of health or chronic disease. Scientists have studied populations all over the globe and consistently found that the people with the lowest incidence of chronic disease and the longest life spans eat a traditional whole-food, plant-based diet naturally rich in starchy vegetables and containing an abundance of vitamins, minerals, enzymes, antioxidants, and phytonutrients. Most traditional/ancestral diets are low in animal products and contain no processed food. And we know from the National Geographic Society's Blue Zones project that the longest-living populations around the world on every continent eat diets that are on average about 95 percent plant based. That equates to eating animal products somewhere between a few times per week and a few times per month. If you live and eat the way the healthy longest-living people live and eat, you can expect to enjoy health and long life free from most chronic diseases everyone else gets.

TAKE OUT
THE TRASH

Garbage in, garbage out.

— ANONYMOUS

YOUR LIVER IS YOUR BODY'S DETOXIFICATION ENGINE and a critical component of your immune system. It processes nearly every toxin that enters your body. An overburdened, sick liver can lead to a toxic body, weakened immune system, and an environment where cancer cells can thrive. So it makes sense to reduce the workload on your liver and the rest of your body by reducing or eliminating your exposure to unnecessary toxins. The overwhelming awareness of how much potentially toxic stuff is around you may induce some anxiety and paranoia at first, but don't let fear take over and paralyze you; just make a to-do list and start cleaning up your life. The goal is to reduce your toxic load, and every little bit helps.

First, you must understand that your body is always detoxifying. Your body detoxifies when you pee, poop, and sweat and every time you exhale. And your body is able to detoxify much faster when you stop polluting it. Cigarettes are the number one cause of cancer. If you smoke, stop smoking. Although e-cigarettes, aka "vaping," are less toxic than tobacco, they still increase your risk of cancer.[1] Flex your determination muscle and break your nicotine addiction. You're better off without it.

If you're eating a Western diet, you're eating a lot of toxic stuff. Artificial additives, preservatives, flavors, colors, sweeteners, and trans fats are all man-made chemicals that you were never meant to ingest. Eliminating processed food and switching to an organic whole-foods, plant-based diet are critical steps in reducing your toxic load and restoring your health. If you are eating conventionally grown produce, you are ingesting trace amounts of toxic pesticides, herbicides, and fungicides that are sprayed on crops. Switching to an all-organic diet (as much as possible) is the first way you can reduce your body's toxic load. The less work your liver has to do to detoxify avoidable toxins, the more bandwidth it has to detoxify the unavoidable ones.

In 2013, researchers at MIT published a study demonstrating that Monsanto's Roundup—the most popular herbicide in the world, sprayed on genetically modified and conventionally grown (non-organic) crops—leaves glyphosate residue, especially on sugar, corn, soy, and wheat. According to their findings, glyphosate interferes with cytochrome P450 enzymes that help your body detoxify. Inhibited detoxification can enhance the damaging effects of other food-borne chemicals and environmental toxins, leading to diabetes, heart disease, autism, cancer, infertility, and more.[2] Glyphosate is also a xenoestrogen, an endocrine disrupter found to promote hormone-dependent breast cancer growth.[3] Internal FDA emails obtained by *The Guardian* through the Freedom of Information Act revealed that one researcher found traces of glyphosate in all the food he brought from home to test except for broccoli, which included wheat crackers, granola, and cornmeal.[4] Glyphosate has also been found in a variety of cereals, chips, crackers, cookies, and even wine and orange juice. This chemical is so widely used that it has polluted our rainwater, groundwater, and drinking water.

Each year the Environmental Working Group publishes a report of the most pesticide-contaminated produce. The rankings are based on the pesticide levels in washed produce reported by the FDA and the USDA Pesticide Testing Program. According to its findings, you can lower your pesticide exposure by nearly 80 percent simply by avoiding the top 12 most contaminated fruits and vegetables, known as the Dirty Dozen.

A study published in the *Journal of Environmental Research* found that after just seven days on an organic diet, dialkyl phosphate pesticide (DAP) levels in adults dropped by 89 percent in urinary excretion. DAPs make up 70 to 80 percent of organophosphate pesticides.[5] In a similar study, researchers also reported a dramatic drop in the levels of insecticides and herbicide in children's urine after only five days on an organic diet.[6]

Produce you should buy organic:

Apples, celery, cherry tomatoes, cucumbers, grapes, hot peppers, nectarines, peaches, potatoes, spinach, strawberries, sweet bell peppers, kale, collard greens, summer squash, corn, and berries.

Produce that isn't critical to buy organic:

Asparagus, avocados, cabbage, cantaloupe, eggplant, grapefruit, honeydew, kiwi, mangoes, mushrooms, onions, papayas (avoid Hawaiian papayas; they are genetically modified), pineapples, sweet peas, sweet potatoes, and watermelons.

The most effective fruit and vegetable wash for pesticide removal appears to be a 10 percent solution of salt water, 1 part salt to 9 parts water.[7]

CHECK THE LABEL

Conventional produce has a four-digit SKU on the sticker starting with a 3 or 4. Organic produce will have a five-digit SKU starting with the number 9. Genetically modified produce typically has a five-digit SKU starting with the number 8, but since it is not required by law, some GMO producers have dropped the 8 and shortened their SKUs to four digits.

If you can't afford or don't have access to organic produce, you should still eat tons of fruits and vegetables. The benefits of the abundance of vitamins, minerals, antioxidants, enzymes, and phytonutrients in a diet rich in fruits and vegetables outweigh any risk.

THE SOLUTION TO POLLUTION IS DILUTION

Our bodies are roughly 60 percent water. Water is the most critical element in your body. Depending on your metabolism and how much body fat you have, you can go anywhere from many weeks to many months without food, but you can only live a week or two without water. Water (hydrogen and oxygen) is essential to life and every system in the body, especially for flushing out toxins.

TIP:
Produce with thin skin is more apt to absorb pesticides than produce with thicker skin. A good rule of thumb if money is tight: If you eat the skin, buy organic. If you don't eat the skin, conventional may be okay.

This is why it is vitally important to put clean water in your body. And lots of it. Half a gallon of purified water per day is ideal (juice counts toward this). Although tap water is relatively clean, and is certainly an improvement over drinking sugary drinks, it still can contain hundreds of contaminants, including lead, copper, bacteria, industrial waste chemicals, and sewage. And even if your tap water is 100 percent contaminant free, it still likely contains chlorine bleach and fluoride. Chlorine bleach is added to kill bacteria, which is good. But then you end up drinking the bleach, which is bad. Fluoride is added to our drinking water for our teeth, but the fluoride used is not naturally sourced or pharmaceutical grade.

Cities with fluoridated water have higher cavity rates and higher cancer death rates than cities with non-fluoridated water. Ninety-eight percent of Western Europe now has rejected water fluoridation, and their children's teeth are just as healthy as children's teeth in the United States. Since 1997, the FDA has required all fluoride toothpaste sold in the United States to carry this poison warning:

Keep out of reach of children under 6 years of age. If you accidentally swallow more than used for brushing, seek professional help or call a poison control center immediately.

This is because a tube of toothpaste contains enough fluoride to kill a small child, and it's not uncommon for young children to swallow some toothpaste while brushing. But even if you don't swallow your toothpaste, fluoride is still absorbed directly into your bloodstream through the capillaries under your tongue.

Roughly 66 percent of U.S. water supplies are currently fluoridated and 90 percent of these municipalities use hydrofluorosilicic acid,[8] a waste product from phosphate fertilizer manufacturing that is often contaminated with arsenic, heavy metals, and radionuclides. Since 1999, over 60 U.S. communities have rejected fluoridation.

Fluoride is an ingredient in some prescription drugs, including Paxil, Prozac, Flonase, and Flovent. Most commercial crops are watered with fluoridated water and absorb it. Fruit juices from concentrate are reconstituted with fluoridated water. And bottled water, even if it's filtered, usually has fluoride in it, unless it's true spring water. Bottled water companies are not required to disclose what type of filtration they use, if any. And don't believe the "natural mountain spring" hype; many companies are simply selling tap water that may be further contaminated by hormone-disrupting chemicals leached from the plastic bottle. A 2018 study found that 93 percent of bottled water brands tested were contaminated with as much as 10,000 plastic microparticles per liter. Nestlé Pure Life bottled water had the highest levels.[9]

Cooking with tap water is also problematic because it concentrates the fluoride and other pollutants, some of which bind to the vegetables you're about to eat. Steaming is the best way to preserve nutrients in vegetables, but if you're going to boil veggies, make sure you use purified water and save the broth for soup stock.

MEET THE HALIDES: UNINVITED GUESTS IN YOUR BODY

Many people have thyroid problems today due to fluoride, chlorine, and bromine. These three toxic halides all displace iodine in the thyroid, essentially polluting it and eventually impairing its ability to function properly. The thyroid regulates your endocrine system, directly affecting breast, ovarian, uterine, and prostate health. Fluoride and chlorine are in our drinking and bathing water and most beverages sold today. Bromine is a flame retardant used to treat furniture, mattresses, and carpet to help keep them from catching fire. Bromine is also used in processed foods in the form of brominated vegetable oil and potassium bromate, as well as in prescription medications.

TIP:
Your body absorbs chlorine when you shower. Invest in a shower filter to remove chlorine from your shower water.

Brominated vegetable oil (BVO) is banned in over 100 countries (but not the U.S.) and is most commonly found in soft drinks and sports drinks like Gatorade, Powerade, Mountain Dew, Squirt, and Fresca. BVO has been linked to major organ system damage, hormone disruption, thyroid dysfunction, birth defects, brain development and growth problems in children, schizophrenia, hearing loss, and cancers of the breast, thyroid, stomach, ovaries, uterus, and prostate. In early 2013, due to public pressure, Pepsi agreed to remove BVO from Gatorade.

Potassium bromate (bromated flour) is used in many baked goods to speed up the baking process. It bleaches the dough and makes it unnaturally white and fluffy—think Wonder Bread. In the early 1980s, Japanese researchers began publishing studies showing that potassium bromate caused thyroid, kidney, and other cancers in rodents. Many countries other than the U.S., including the E.U., China, and Brazil, took these studies seriously and banned potassium bromate in food. The state of California requires a disclosure on food labels that contain it, which says, "Potassium bromate is an unnecessary and potentially harmful food additive, and should be avoided."

TOXIC MEAT AND DAIRY

Meat and dairy can harbor viruses, bacteria, and parasites, and factory-farmed animals are often injected with antibiotics and hormones and are fed unnatural GMO feed to fatten them up. Many wild fish are polluted with mercury, especially the fish at the top of the food chain, including tuna, tilefish, swordfish, shark, and king mackerel. On the other hand, farm-raised fish have been found to have some of the highest levels of PCBs, a toxic by-product of the manufacturing industry. Dairy, eggs, and meat also have been found to concentrate environmental toxins and pesticide residues in their fatty tissues.[10]

Aluminum is a potent neurotoxin linked to Alzheimer's.[11] You might be surprised to know that the highest source of dietary aluminum is cheese. Many cheese manufacturers use an additive called sodium aluminum phosphate, which is a form of salt that enhances flavor and texture. But you won't see sodium aluminum phosphate listed as an ingredient on the label because cheese makers are allowed to simply call it "salt." Other forms of aluminum, such as aluminum sulfate, are often used in baking powders, pickles, relishes, flour, and canned meat. The half-life of mercury in the body is estimated to be about two months. The same goes for aluminum. Your body can remove these heavy metals, but you have to stop putting them in.

The most important steps in detoxification are to stop putting toxins in your mouth via drinking, smoking, and eating man-made processed food and animal products, as well as prescription drugs (consult your doctor before stopping them).

TOXIC BEAUTY

Your skin absorbs what you put on it. Chemicals from creams, lotions, potions, oils, makeup, nail polish, deodorants, and other body care products are absorbed into your bloodstream through your skin, and these chemicals circulate throughout your entire body. Unlike the food industry, the skin care industry is largely unregulated. Mascara has traces of mercury. Lipstick has traces of lead. Talcum powder has been associated with ovarian cancer. According to a study conducted by the Organic Consumers Association, traces of suspected carcinogen 1,4-dioxane were found in almost half of personal care products tested, even though it is typically not listed on the label.[12] This included bath products, shower gels, lotions, and hand soaps. Aluminum salts in antiperspirants, which interfere with estrogen receptors, have been implicated as a potential contributor to breast cancer, as there is a disproportionately large number of breast cancers that occur in the upper outer quadrant of the breast tissue closest to the armpit.[13]

The Environmental Working Group website (ewg.org) has a large database of body care products rated by toxicity. It's a great place to research the brands you're using to see if they are potentially toxic and to find top-rated, clean brands.

Toxic Body Care Chemicals to Avoid

Here is a selected list of toxic chemicals commonly used in personal care products that you should steer clear of, courtesy of the Environmental Working Group.

1. **BHA** (butylated hydroxyanisole) is a suspected human carcinogen found in food, food packaging, and personal care products sold in the U.S. In animal studies, BHA produces liver damage and causes stomach cancers (such as papillomas and carcinomas) and interferes with reproductive system development and thyroid function (hormone levels). The European Union considers it unsafe in fragrance.

2. **Coal tar** and other coal tar ingredients (aminophenol, diaminobenzene, phenylenediamine) are used in hair dyes and specialty products such as dandruff and psoriasis shampoos. Coal tar is a known human carcinogen. Hair stylists and other professionals are exposed to these chemicals in hair dye almost daily and have a higher risk of cancer than many other professions. Europe has banned the use of many of these coal tar ingredients in hair dyes.

3. **Formaldehyde and formaldehyde releasers** (bronopol, DMDM hydantoin, diazolidinyl urea, imidzaolidinyl urea, and quaternium-15). Formaldehyde is a preservative and a known human carcinogen as well as an asthmagen, neurotoxicant, and developmental toxicant. It is used in hair straighteners and as a preservative in cosmetics. Formaldehyde releasers are widely used in U.S. products. Not surprisingly, more Americans develop contact allergies to these ingredients than Europeans. Also, the artificial sweetener aspartame breaks down into formaldehyde in the body.

4. **Fragrances** is the generic catch-all term used to avoid disclosing secret ingredients to competitors, but it's also

a way to hide potentially toxic ingredients. Federal law doesn't require companies to list any of the chemicals in their fragrance mixture on their product labels. Recent research from EWG and the Campaign for Safe Cosmetics found an average of 14 chemicals in 17 name-brand fragrance products, none of them listed on the label. Fragrances can contain hormone disruptors and are among the top five allergens in the world. I recommend buying fragrance free or from companies that provide full label disclosure.

5. **Parabens** (specifically propyl-, isopropyl-, butyl-, and isobutyl-parabens) are estrogen-mimicking preservatives used widely in cosmetics and body care products like shampoos and conditioners. Parabens may disrupt the endocrine system and cause reproductive and developmental disorders.

6. **Polyethylene glycol (PEGs) and other polyethylene compounds** are a family of conditioning and cleaning agents that go by many names. These synthetic chemicals are frequently contaminated with 1,4-dioxane, which the U.S. government considers a probable human carcinogen and which readily penetrates the skin.

7. **Petroleum distillates** are petroleum-extracted cosmetics ingredients, commonly found in mascara. They may cause contact dermatitis and are often contaminated with cancer-causing impurities. They are produced in oil refineries at the same time as automobile fuel, heating oil, and chemical feedstocks.

8. **Phthalates** are found in color cosmetics, fragranced lotions, body washes, hair care products, nail polish, and more. They can cause endocrine disruption, developmental and reproductive toxicity, organ system toxicity, and bioaccumulation of toxic substances. Pregnant women and breast-feeding mothers are especially vulnerable. Phthalates are banned from cosmetics sold in the E.U. but not in the U.S. Look for phthalate-free brands and avoid products with "fragrance," which may contain phthalates.

9. **Resorcinol** is a common ingredient in hair color and bleaching products. It is a skin irritant, toxic to the immune system, and a frequent cause of hair dye allergy. In animal studies resorcinol has been shown to disrupt normal thyroid function.

10. **Triclosan and triclocarban** are antimicrobial pesticides found in antibacterial soaps. Triclosan disrupts thyroid function and reproductive hormones. Overuse may promote the development of bacterial resistance. These chemicals are highly toxic to the aquatic environment. Colgate made national headlines in 2014 when it was discovered that Colgate Total toothpaste contained triclosan.

11. **Vitamin A compounds** (retinol, retinyl palmitate, retinyl acetate) are widely used in sunscreens, skin lotions, lip products, and makeup. Sunlight breaks down vitamin A to produce toxic free radicals that can damage DNA and hasten skin lesions and tumors in lab animals.

A CANCER CAUSE RIGHT UNDER YOUR NOSE

If you have cancer, the cause could literally be right under your nose, in your mouth, specifically from silver fillings. Silver amalgam fillings are 50 percent mercury, the most toxic nonradioactive metal on earth. Silver fillings release mercury vapor every time you agitate your teeth with chewing, brushing, eating acidic foods, and drinking hot liquids. Your body absorbs 80 percent of the mercury vapor you breathe in. Each amalgam in your mouth can release as much as 1 microgram of mercury per day, and the release of mercury vapor never stops, no matter how old the fillings are. Tests have found that people with silver fillings have mercury circulating in their blood, brain, liver, kidneys, and even amniotic fluid and breast milk. Because of the excessive use of mercury fillings, it is estimated that over 120 million Americans have mercury exposure that exceeds the safety limit set by the

California Environmental Protection Agency.[14] If you have two or more mercury fillings, you are probably in that group. (For more information, visit the International Academy of Oral Medicine and Toxicology at iaomt.org.)

The American Dental Association's official position is that mercury amalgams are safe. Mercury amalgams were first introduced into dentistry in the early 1800s, long before safety regulations were enacted. Today the EPA and OSHA classify mercury filings as hazardous waste, requiring strict disposal procedures to prevent further release of mercury into the environment after fillings are removed from dental patients' mouths.

If you decide to have your mercury fillings replaced, avoid bisphenol-A based epoxy resin composites. The New England Children's Amalgam Trial linked these types of resins to a greater risk of impaired physiological function in children, including learning impairment and behavioral issues. Make sure your dentist uses a non–BPA-based composite resin for your fillings.

The half-life of mercury in the body is estimated to be about two months.[15] If mercury exposure from sources like fish and silver fillings is stopped, it is estimated that the body can almost completely detoxify mercury within a year. Oral DMSA (dimercaptosuccinic acid) therapy is a mercury and lead detoxification protocol that may accelerate the process. This should only be done under the supervision of a qualified practitioner.

MERCURY IN OUR FOOD

Mercury has made its way into our food supply. Almost all fish and shellfish contain trace amounts of mercury in their bodies, trapped in their fatty tissue. Like polonium, mercury works its way up the food chain in a process called biomagnification. The bigger the fish and the longer it lives, the more toxic mercury it absorbs, and when you eat that fish you absorb it all and it accumulates in your tissues. The human body can detoxify mercury but it can take many months, and consistent mercury exposure over time can lead to a toxic buildup and eventual tipping point when your body's ability to repair, regenerate, and detoxify properly is compromised, its functions break down, and health problems begin.

Mercury consumption from fish has been linked to brain and nervous system damage in unborn babies and young children, which is why the FDA and EPA strongly advise that women who are pregnant, may become pregnant, breast-feeding mothers, and young children abstain from fish known to have high levels of mercury, such as tuna, tilefish, king mackerel, marlin, orange roughy, shark, and swordfish. Mercury poisons adults too. In 1969 the FDA determined that 0.5 ppm was the maximum allowable limit for mercury in fish, but mercury levels in fish kept rising. So in 1979 they raised the limit to 1 ppm. In 1984 they stopped measuring total mercury and decided to only check for methylmercury. In 1998 the FDA stopped widely testing for mercury in fish. To put it in perspective, eating mercury-containing fish like tuna just once per week may exceed the EPA safety level and expose you to more mercury than six thimerosal-containing vaccines.

MY MERCURY EXPOSURE

When I was in fourth grade, I got a fever and stayed home sick from school. While playing with the dog in the living room with a thermometer in my mouth, I hit my chin on the coffee table, biting the glass thermometer in half. This was a fairly common problem with kids and glass thermometers, which is why they don't sell them anymore. Years later when I was a junior in high school, I thought it would be cool to "accidentally" break a huge thermometer on the lab table in chemistry class. I poured some of the mercury into the palm of my hand and let it roll around for a few seconds. I remember one of the other kids saying, "I don't think you're supposed to touch that stuff." At which point I let it roll off my hand back onto the table. Holding mercury in my hand was strange because it was surprisingly heavy, like a liquid marble. When I was diagnosed with colon cancer, my doctor estimated it had been growing in my body for about 10 years.

FRESH AIR IS UNDERRATED

An important step to reduce your toxic load is to eliminate as many potential toxins as possible from the two places where you spend most of your time: home and work. A 2018 study published in *Science* found that volatile organic compounds from paint, varnishes, cleaning products, and personal care products including shampoo, hairspray, deodorant, perfume, air fresheners, and hand sanitizers contribute to more outdoor air pollution than automobile exhaust.[16] And we spend 90 percent of our time indoors! According to the EPA, indoor air can be as much as five times more polluted than outside air. Common indoor air pollutants also include radon gas, smoke, mold spores, and volatile organic compounds from chemicals used in furniture foam and fabrics. Radon gas is the second leading cause of lung cancer after smoking.[17] You can get a radon gas test kit for $15 at your local hardware store. While you're there, pick up a mold test kit. Toxic mold can lead to chronic infection and suppressed immunity, which can keep you perpetually sick and vulnerable to cancer. Scented candles, incense, and air fresheners can produce toxic chemical vapors and smoke. Look for 100 percent soy or beeswax candles with paper or cotton wicks scented with essential oils. Diffusing essential oils is also a safer option, but certain oils can be toxic to pets.

Air purifiers can help clean up the air in your home and so can houseplants. Multiple studies have found that houseplants remove common indoor air pollutants, such as benzene, trichloroethylene, formaldehyde, and ammonia. Some of the best performers are peace lily, Boston fern, bamboo palm, lady palm, Barberton daisy, mass cane, Janet Craig, and warneckei. For optimal air filtering, NASA recommends one plant for every 100 square feet of indoor space.[18,19] Note: Before you bring new plants into the house, make sure they aren't toxic to pets.

CLEAN UP YOUR CLEANING SUPPLIES

Many household cleaning products contain noxious and toxic ingredients than can be absorbed through your skin and when you inhale the fumes. An eight-year study following over 55,000 American nurses reported that nurses who used disinfectants to clean surfaces at least once a week had a 24 to 32 percent increased risk of developing chronic obstructive pulmonary disease, emphysema, bronchitis, and asthma when compared to nurses who used disinfectants less frequently.[20] The main cleaning chemicals linked to lung damage in the study were glutaraldehyde, a disinfectant used on medical instruments, as well as bleach, hydrogen peroxide, alcohol, and ammonia-based compounds, which are commonly found in household cleaners.

A 2018 study out of Norway found that women who reported using cleaning products at least once per week in their home or cleaned professionally for 20 years had substantial lung damage, equivalent to smoking 20 cigarettes per day, compared to women who didn't clean their own homes.[21] Women who cleaned for a living had the most damage and the highest decline in lung function. To prevent lung damage from harsh cleaning chemicals, the scientists who conducted the research advise using microfiber cloths and water instead of harsh chemical cleaning products.

Even laundry detergents and dryer sheets can be polluting your home. An analysis of gases produced by household laundry machines found more than 25 volatile organic compounds, including seven hazardous air pollutants, such as known carcinogens acetaldehyde and benzene.[22]

I recommend replacing standard chemical household cleaners, laundry detergent, and especially dish detergent with natural, nontoxic, biodegradable, organic cleaning products. Dr. Bronner's Pure Castile Soap is one of our favorites. You can use it in the shower. You can do your dishes with it. You can clean your house with it. You can even brush your teeth with it.

IS YOUR JOB TOXIC?

In 2009 an occupational study of cancer risk for 15 million people from Denmark, Finland, Iceland, Norway, and Sweden found the highest risk of cancer in beverage and tobacco workers, plumbers, seamen, mechanics, engine operators, miners, chimney sweeps, and some factory workers. These professions involve working around smoke, soot, dust, or chemical fumes. Hair stylists and salon workers also have elevated risk due to their exposure to chemical agents in hair care products like straighteners, bleaches, dyes, perfumes, and nail polish. Restaurant servers have an elevated risk of lung cancer from tobacco use and exposure, as well as liver cancer from alcohol use.[23] According to the study, the occupations with the lowest risk for cancer are farmers, gardeners, and teachers. But it's a different story for livestock producers. Multiple studies have linked American poultry, cattle, and pig farmers to elevated risk of blood cancers.[24,25]

Detoxifying your workplace can be tricky. Unless you're the boss, you may not be able to improve the air quality at work. Adding several small plants, or even a desktop air purifier, in your office or cubicle can help. If you are surrounded by toxic fumes at work, it might be a good time to start looking for another job.

ELECTROPOLLUTION

Your body is an electrically powered organic machine, and your cells communicate with each other through electrical impulses. Your brain tells your heart to beat. Your stomach tells your brain you are hungry. Your skin sends information to your brain about the texture, temperature, and weight of objects you touch, and so much more.

Your central nervous system is kind of like the internet. It is the conduit for trillions of messages to be sent back and forth between your cells, organs, and brain to keep your body functioning properly. When you cut yourself, distress signals are sent out by the wounded area and your body responds with reinforcements to clot the blood, fight infection, seal off the area, and rebuild the damaged tissue.

When electrical current flows through an object, it creates an electromagnetic field (EMF), and just like electrical wiring and electronic equipment, our bodies have an electromagnetic field surrounding them. We conduct electricity and radio frequencies, which is why getting close to or touching the TV antenna can affect the picture. Our bodies run on electricity, but not all electricity is good for us.

Electropollution is a term coined to describe our increasing exposure to harmful invisible electronic frequencies harnessed by man in our modern world. Electronic frequency can be divided into these basic groups:

➤ **Extremely low frequency (ELF):** power lines

➤ **Radio frequency (RF):** radio and TV signals, microwaves, and wireless devices

➤ **Intermediate frequencies:** emitted by appliances and electric circuits

➤ **High frequency:** ionizing radiation, X-rays, CT scans, and PET scans

➤ **Dirty electricity:** the harmful combination of distorted frequencies from various electronic sources in our homes, offices, schools, and elsewhere

According to the research and hypothesis of Samuel Milham, M.D., M.P.H., the widespread adoption of electricity in our homes, which was completed in 1959, is correlated to the rise in cancer, cardiovascular disease, diabetes, and even suicide in the United States. The incidence of these diseases was much lower in rural areas before they were electrified, and there was a distinct increase in the years following electrification.[26] In 1979 a study by Leeper and Wertheimer was published showing a correlation between living in close proximity to strong magnetic fields emitted by residential power lines and risk of childhood cancer.[27] Since then additional studies have also shown an increase in cancer risk while others have shown no increase in risk. Two pooled studies and a meta-analysis found a 1.4 to 2-fold increase in risk of leukemia in children exposed to electromagnetic fields at home measuring 0.3 μT or higher. However, according to the National Cancer Institute, the number of children exposed to this level of electromagnetic fields in the combined studies is considered to be too small to be statistically significant. Given the lack of conclusive evidence either way, I think it makes sense to follow the precautionary principle and take steps to reduce your exposure to potentially harmful electromagnetic frequencies. Not living next to power lines is a good start.

The microwave frequencies produced by 2.4 GHz Wi-Fi devices have been identified as an important threat to human health. Numerous repeated studies have linked Wi-Fi radiation to oxidative stress, DNA damage, hormone dysregulation, melatonin lowering and sleep disruption, infant brain development, calcium overload, and male infertility.[28]

If you're living near an industrial area, you could be exposed to higher levels of air and water pollution. And there may be significant pollution nearby that you aren't aware of. I suggest researching to see if there are any EPA superfund sites in your area. These are known toxic-waste hazard sites across the United States (https://www.epa.gov/superfund). Also check to see if you live in a cancer cluster, which is an area known to have higher than average rates of cancer. Deaths from all cancers in 2014 were highest along the Mississippi River, near the Kentucky/West Virginia border, in western Alaska, and in the South in general. Cancer deaths were lowest in western states like Utah and Colorado.[29] If you live in an area with high rates of cancer, if multiple neighbors are getting cancer, or if more than one person in your house is diagnosed with cancer, you may need to get the heck out of there.

How to Reduce Harmful EMF Exposure in Your Home

➤ Just like light, EMFs can also interfere with your body's production of melatonin. Don't charge your cell phone on the nightstand beside your bed.

➤ Turn off your Wi-Fi at night or when you aren't using it. Newer wireless routers have on/off switches for the Wi-Fi signal and some can even be controlled with your smartphone. If your wireless router doesn't have an on/off switch, a cheap hack is to plug it into a light timer programmed to shut off automatically at a certain time each night.

➤ Fluorescent bulbs generate more EMFs than standard bulbs, produce harmful blue light, and are filled with toxic mercury vapor. LED light bulbs generate less EMFs but also produce blue light, which you should avoid at night. Incandescent bulbs are best.

➤ If you would like to measure the EMF fields in your home or at work, you can use a gauss meter to measure EMF "hot spots" in your home or work environment so you can take steps to reduce your exposure.

Your cells are constantly sending and receiving messages via electrochemical pathways in your nervous system, but external electromagnetic frequencies can disrupt normal communication between cells. They can overload and confuse cells with false messages or messages they don't understand, like when too many people try to talk at the same time. This interference can disrupt cellular function in every part of your body. When you are exposed to harmful EMFs, they can disturb your nervous system and raise your stress hormones, which can lead to sleep disorders, depressed immunity, cardiovascular disease, premature aging, autoimmune disorders, and even neurological problems like depression. Harmful EMFs can rupture cell membranes and create free radicals, resulting in DNA damage. They can disrupt normal cell division, handicap your immune system, and create precancerous cells. If you have health problems, electropollution is not likely to be something your doctor is going to consider but it could be aggravating or even causing your condition.

WHAT ABOUT CELL PHONE RADIATION?

If cell phone radiation causes brain cancer, then it stands to reason that the widespread adoption of cell phones starting in the early 1990s should have caused a measurable increase in the number of new brain cancers diagnosed each year. However, data from the National Cancer Institute's SEER Program shows no increase in the incidence of brain or other central nervous system cancers between 1992 and 2015, despite the dramatic increase in cell phone use in the United States during this time.[30]

But these stats don't tell the whole story. According to a 2018 UK study, the rates of several types of brain cancers have fallen, but the overall annual incidence of glioblastoma multiforme, the most aggressive type of brain cancer, has doubled since 1995.[31] The authors of the study speculate that this could be due to increased exposure to factors such as medical X-rays and CT scans, pollution, or cell phone radiation.

The World Health Organization's International Agency for Research on Cancer has classified cell phone use as "possibly carcinogenic to humans," but along with the American Cancer Society, the National Institute of Environmental Health Sciences, as well as the FDA, CDC, and FCC, the IARC also states that there is not enough evidence to conclusively link cell phone use to brain tumors.

Given the lack of conclusive evidence concerning cell phones and cancer risk, I still think it makes sense to take precautions. I rarely if ever put my phone up to my head. I always try to use the speaker phone or earbuds, and I keep my phone away from my body whenever possible. I put my phone on my desk when

I'm working, on the table at restaurants, or in the console when I'm driving. I also put my phone on airplane mode for hours at a time, especially if it's in my pocket for long periods of time. When using your phone, be aware that the weaker your phone's signal, the more radiation it emits.

FASTING

Fasting was a regular part of life for many of our ancestors for religious reasons and during times of food scarcity. And it is a powerful detoxification method and regeneration therapy for your body. I fasted often during my cancer healing journey and did several extended-day juice fasts, drinking only vegetable juice for up to 10 days as well as taking shorter water fasts.

Fasting gives your body a break from digestion, which allows it to pay attention to things that have been overlooked. Around day two or three of a water fast, your body switches from burning glucose for energy to burning body fat. This process is called ketosis. When you enter a natural state of ketosis through fasting, which is technically controlled starvation, your body switches from normal daily operations to survival and protection mode and your cells begin a process of internal housecleaning. Realizing there is a shortage of glucose for fuel, healthy cells stop trying to grow and instead begin to break down and use old and damaged parts for fuel. The scientific term for this is autophagy, which is derived from Greek and means "self-eating." During this process, healthy cells "hunker down" and reinforce their defenses to protect themselves and survive, but cancer cells are mutated cells stuck in growth mode and have difficulty adapting. During a period of fasting or starvation, many types of cancer cells keep trying to grow without fuel and become weaker and die.

Sometimes cells live too long and become old and ineffective. These are not the kinds of cells you want in your body, especially when it comes to your immune cells. During a three- to five-day water fast, old and damaged immune cells in your body die off and regenerative stem cells are activated. Then when you start eating again, these activated stem cells ramp up production of brand-new immune cells to replace the old ones that died off.[32] Fasting essentially reboots and recharges your immune system and reduces levels of IGF-1, insulin, and glucose in your body.

Researchers have even found that short-term fasting protects healthy cells and sensitizes cancer cells to chemo and radiotherapy treatment in mice, extending their survival.[33] Fasting for 72 hours around cancer treatment—48 hours before and 24 hours after—has been determined to be safe for cancer patients and to reduce the side effects of platinum combination chemotherapy while protecting healthy cells.[34]

The guidelines for fasting are simple. Drink water throughout the day; somewhere between half and one gallon is sufficient. You can squeeze lemon into your water and drink non-caffeinated herbal teas like rooibos or hibiscus. Taking supplements may be okay too. There aren't enough calories in lemon juice, teas, or supplements to interfere with the process. Most people can handle a three- to five-day water fast without any problems, but under certain conditions—like if you are taking drugs that lower blood pressure or blood sugar—fasting could be dangerous. If you are taking pharmaceutical drugs or have any serious health conditions or concerns, you should check with your doctor before attempting a water fast.

An alternative to water fasting is the ProLon Fasting Mimicking Diet developed by Dr. Valter Longo, director of the Longevity Institute at the University of Southern California. The Fasting Mimicking Diet is a five-day, plant-based, calorie-restricted meal plan that has been proven in human clinical trials to produce the same powerful benefits in the body as a water fast, including autophagy and stem cell activation and regeneration.[35] My wife and I have done the ProLon Diet. It is easier than a water fast because you don't have to stop eating completely, and it may be safer for individuals with serious health conditions. For maximum physiological benefit, Dr. Longo recommends doing this diet once per month for three months in a row, and then once per quarter or every six months. He and his team are currently conducting clinical trials examining the extent to which a fasting mimicking diet protects healthy cells and enhances conventional cancer treatments.

It's normal to feel lousy during the first few days of a fast. This is known as the Herxheimer Reaction, or the "healing crisis." You may even experience this just by converting from a Western diet to a raw-food or plant-based diet. There are three main reasons why: adaptation, food addiction, and detoxification. During fasting, your body flips genetic survival switches that it has never flipped before and that's going to make you feel different. Most people are adapted to a diet that is high in animal protein and fat, sugar, salt, and caffeine. When you remove these things from your diet, you will experience physical withdrawal. If you have been in the habit of drinking diet sodas or chewing gum all day, you may also suffer withdrawal from food additives like aspartame.

The second reason you may feel bad when you fast or switch to a raw-food or a plant-based diet is the detoxification reaction. Your body stores toxins in fat. And during a fast, your body will break down toxic fat for energy. Some of these toxins are released into your bloodstream and circulate throughout your body before they are neutralized and eliminated. During this process, you're going to feel lousy. Some typical reactions caused by the adaptation process, food withdrawal, or detoxification are low energy, brain fog, headaches, dizziness, nausea, random aches and pains, pimples, rashes, and upset stomach. Every person has a different experience. In some cases, it could even trigger a fever, which could be beneficial. Your immune system ramps up into high gear when you have a fever, and a fever can wipe out a host of viruses, bacteria, and parasites in your body that you didn't even know you had. Note: If you develop a fever over 104°F, call your doctor and discontinue the fast.

If any of those reactions happen during a fast, it could be coincidental, but it's likely because there's some serious housecleaning happening in your body. Make sure you are super hydrated. Drink lots of water to help flush things out and power through it if you can. A water enema or a quick sweat in a sauna—20 minutes or less—can also help accelerate detoxification. Note: If you're taking prescription medication, fasting and/or saunas could be dangerous. Make sure that you are cautious with your approach and do it with supervision—medical, if necessary.

The typical scenario during a fast is low energy, and maybe a bit of a headache for a few days. If you start feeling bad, just remind yourself that it is part of the process. Most folks feel okay on day one, lousy and hungry on day two, and then turn a corner and lose their appetite and start to feel good on day three. When you get over that detoxification hump, usually after a few days, you should feel great. Every time I fast, there's always a point around day three of the fast where I am surprised at how much energy I have and how good I feel without being hungry.

A 24-hour water fast is an easy way to get your feet wet. However, a three-day water fast is considered to be the minimal length of time needed to get the benefits of autophagy and stem cell regeneration. If you are doing a three-day fast, I recommend doing it over a weekend. Start on a Friday morning—Thursday night would be your last meal—and don't eat again until Monday morning.

Most folks lose 1 to 2 pounds per day during a fast, but some of the weight returns once you resume eating. Fasting can jump-start weight loss, but the best way to lose weight and keep it off is by consistently eating a whole-food, plant-based diet. The more body fat you have, the longer you can fast. Obesity is the second leading cause of cancer, and getting rid of excess body fat is a very good thing. The powerful regenerative effects of fasting actually happen after the fast, when you resume eating after fasting for three to five days.

MASSIVE ACTION STEPS FOR DETOXIFICATION

➤ Stop putting artificial food loaded with man-made chemicals in your mouth

➤ Stop eating animal foods

➤ Buy organic produce

➤ Invest in a water purifier and a filter for your shower

➤ Replace your toxic makeup and body care with non-toxic brands

➤ Remove mercury fillings

➤ Keep your cell phone away from your head

➤ Turn off Wi-Fi at night and whenever possible

➤ Invest in an air purifier

➤ Replace your toxic cleaning supplies

➤ Consider a three- to five-day water fast or the ProLon five-day Fasting Mimicking Diet

LET'S GET PHYSICAL

Those who think they have not time for bodily exercise
will sooner or later have to find time for illness.

— EDWARD STANLEY, EARL OF DERBY

If you can't fly, run. If you can't run, walk. If you can't walk, crawl.
But by all means, keep moving.

— DR. MARTIN LUTHER KING, JR.

MANY PEOPLE ASSUME that health and fitness are synonymous, because typically when someone decides to get fit they start working out, eating better, and losing weight, and subsequently their health improves. But it is possible to be fit and unhealthy. It is also possible to be perfectly healthy but not very strong or fit. The goal is to achieve a balance of both. It's not unusual for athletes and fitness buffs to become so obsessed with performance and their physical appearance that they will put anything in their bodies to achieve their goals. Many eat large amounts of animal protein and take copious amounts of sports supplements and growth hormones to get big and ripped, or stronger and faster. Cancer survivor Mr. Livestrong himself, Lance Armstrong, admitted to using illegal drugs to win the Tour de France.

SITTING IS THE NEW SMOKING

Americans have become sedentary beings who spend on average 15.5 of our 16 to 17 waking hours per day sitting, and one-third of American children and two-thirds of American adults are either overweight or obese. According to recent estimates, half of Americans don't get enough physical activity, and over one-third of us are classified as "physically inactive." Lack of exercise is a major contributor to chronic diseases including cardiovascular diseases, diabetes, breast cancer, colon cancer, and endometrial cancer and increases your risk of 10 more cancers.[1,2] But you can reduce your risk by simply adding a little more movement to your life.

TOO MUCH OF A GOOD THING

Americans have the shortest life expectancies of any nation in the industrialized world, but professional athletes, who are at the opposite end of the exercise spectrum, have an even shorter life span. The average elite athlete dies by age 67, nine years before the average American coach potato, who has a life expectancy of about 78 (76 for men, 80 for women).

Exercise is definitely a good thing but, extreme exercise, including excessive weight training and endurance training for marathons and triathlons, may do more harm than good. This level of activity can also produce excessive levels of free radicals and high levels of the stress hormones adrenaline and cortisol, which can suppress immune function and raise your risk of infection or illnesses like colds and the flu.

Research done by David Nieman, Ph.D., and colleagues at Loma Linda University showed that marathon runners are six times more likely to become ill after a race due to impaired immune function. Extreme exercise creates excessive catabolic stress and increases the metabolism for prolonged periods of time, increasing free radicals and damaging cells. Marathons and intense aerobic exercise deplete existing antioxidants, suppress immunity, and break down muscle tissue.[3] Chronic physical stress from overtraining week after week, month after month, year after year without adequate recovery time keeps your body in an exhausted, depleted, and vulnerable state.

Exercise alone cannot produce optimal health. Jim Fixx, the "father of jogging" and author of the massive worldwide best-seller *The Complete Book of Running*, died of a heart attack after his morning run at the ripe old age of 52. His autopsy revealed complete blockage in one of his coronary arteries, 80 percent blockage in another, and signs of previous heart attacks.[4] Despite Jim's example and many others, the assumption that fitness equals health is still prevalent today.

Current research indicates that 90 minutes of intense exercise per day, or running 60 miles per week, is too much for most people. Consistent training at this level can keep you in a chronic state of exhaustion, inflammation, and adrenal depletion, all of which elevate your risk for developing disease. This is especially important for cancer patients. Some cancer patients with a strong will to live believe that if they punish their bodies with extreme exercise like long-distance running or triathlons, they are somehow beating back their cancer, but this kind of behavior can have the opposite effect. Extreme exercise creates excessive physical stress on the body that can suppress your immune system for up to 72 hours after each workout, increasing your risk of infections. A 2.5 hour run can drop your natural killer cell count by 50 percent.[5] Extreme exercise can also lead to injury and extended debilitation, during which you lose the benefits of daily exercise.

The internal repair required after extreme exercise can also monopolize valuable resources that the body needs to heal cancer. In addition to suppressing immune function, extreme exercise creates large amounts of lactic acid in the body, which can block key nutrients from reaching healthy cells, and even fuel cancer growth.

THE RIGHT AMOUNT OF EXERCISE

All movement, including light, moderate, and heavy exercise, can be beneficial as long as you get the balance right. For most folks, this means more exercise than you get sitting at a desk all day and less exercise than you would get training for the Olympics. While many people view exercise as a means to get stronger or to look better on the beach, the primary goal of exercise should be to increase your life span and your health span, which is your number of healthy years. Looking better on the beach is a bonus.

Daily moderate aerobic exercise like brisk walking, short running, bike riding, yoga, weight training, and dancing improves immune function by boosting T cell production, increases oxygenation of tissues, improves function of antioxidant enzymes, and triggers the release of endorphins that make you feel good. Exercise has been proven to be an effective antidepressant and to reduce anxiety.[6]

Exercise has also been shown to reverse the loss of muscle tissue and bone mass in cancer patients and the elderly. When you consistently lift heavy weights, you send signals to your body to strengthen your muscles and bones. Routinely lifting heavy weights is the best way to prevent and reverse osteoporosis, far better than taking calcium supplements.

TIP:

If you work out at a public gym, don't touch your eyes, nose, or mouth, and make sure you wash your hands immediately afterward. Gyms are a breeding ground for pathogens and bacteria, which is why my wife and I jokingly refer to the gym as "the germ."

Diet and exercise also affect how your genes express themselves, literally turning good genes on and bad genes off.[7] A Finnish study done on twins showed that exercise reduced mortality by 66 percent for people age 25 to 64, and numerous studies have shown the powerful effect that exercise can have on cancer care and recovery.[8] Breast cancer patients who exercised regularly (the equivalent of walking 30 minutes per day) and ate five or more servings of fruits and vegetables per day had half the recurrence rate after nine years compared to patients who didn't exercise or eat lots of fruits and veggies.[9] That's huge!

Another study found that after moderate- to high-intensity exercise, the blood of breast cancer patients dripped on cancer cells had more cancer stopping power than their pre-exercise blood.[10]

A study published in the *British Medical Journal* found that bicycling to work was associated with a 45 percent reduced risk of dying from cancer and a 46 percent reduced risk of heart disease.[11] There's nothing magic about cycling; it's just that those who rode their bike to work consistently hit the ideal target of health-promoting exercise, which is 30 minutes of moderate to vigorous aerobic exercise per day.

A 2014 study of over 4,600 Swedish men with early stage pros-tate cancer found that the men who engaged in walking or biking every day for 20 minutes or more had a 39 percent lower risk of dying from prostate cancer and a 30 percent lower risk of dying from any other cause compared to the men who were less active.[12]

A 2014 study published in the *Journal of Clinical Oncology* found that colon cancer patients who exercised seven hours per week or more were 31 percent less likely to die from any cause than those who did not exercise at all. The study also found that patients who averaged five hours of TV watching per day were 22 percent more likely to die than those who watched less than two hours per day.[13]

Exercise can reverse decades of damage caused by being sed-entary. In a study of out-of-shape, middle-aged adults, two years of consistent aerobic exercise four to five days per week was found to reverse years of damage, significantly improving their heart health.[14]

Exercise keeps your immune system strong even in old age. Our immune systems decline as we age and as we become less active, which makes us more susceptible to health problems like infections and cancer, but surprising research published in 2018 found that long-distance cyclists in their 60s, 70s, and 80s were found to have the same level of T cells in their blood as people in their 20s![15]

HOW EXERCISE PROMOTES DETOXIFICATION

Every day you are bombarded with toxins in your environment and in your food, which is why detoxification is such a critical process in your body. If the detox process is hindered, toxins can build up, eventually causing acidity and toxemia. A critical component of your immune system hinges on your body's ability to efficiently detoxify via your lymphatic system, which includes your tonsils, thymus, bone marrow, spleen, lymphatic fluid, vessels, and lymph nodes. The thymus and bone marrow produce white blood cells called lymphocytes. Your blood vessels deliver oxygen and nutrients to your cells. Your lymph vessels are like blood vessels and they contain clear lymphatic fluid that carries white blood cells (B cell and T cell lymphocytes) throughout your body to attack invaders and infected cells. Your lymphatic fluid also carries dead cells, metabolic waste, and toxins away from healthy tissue to be eliminated through sweat, mucus, urine, and liver bile, which is carried out in your poop.

Lymph nodes are like holding stations that filter the lymph fluid and capture microbes for B and T cells to deal with. They are located in your armpits, groin, and neck and around the blood vessels of your chest and abdomen. You have about three times more lymphatic fluid than blood, but there's no pump in the lymphatic system. Instead, voluntary and involuntary muscle contractions in your body circulate the lymphatic fluid through a series of one-way valves.

One of the lesser known benefits of exercise is that it moves your lymphatic fluid, promoting detoxification in your body.

The more you move your body, the more you move your lymphatic fluid. When I first started researching, I read every natural cancer survival testimony I could find and I found many common threads, one of which was getting exercise by jumping on a mini-trampoline, aka "rebounding." I figured that since so many natural survivors and health practitioners were recommending it, there must be something to it, so I bought myself a rebounder.

Jumping on a trampoline creates increased G-force resistance (gravitational load) and is thought to positively stress every cell in your body and strengthen your entire musculoskeletal system: your bones, muscles, connective tissue, and even organs. Rebounding promotes lymphatic circulation by stimulating the millions of one-way valves in your lymphatic system. In addition, rebounding is low impact, is gentle on your joints, and improves strength and balance. Rebounding allows you to do jumping and aerobic exercises for much longer intervals than you could on solid ground.

The Three Basic Rebounding Exercises

To do the health bounce, you gently bounce up and down on a rebounder mini-trampoline without your feet leaving the mat. While this may not feel like exercise, it provides enough motion to effectively move your lymphatic system. Many folks can easily do this type of gentle bouncing for 30 minutes to an hour or more, even while watching TV.

The strength bounce involves jumping as high as you can. This movement strengthens primary and stabilizer muscles throughout your body, improves your balance, and moves your lymphatic system. Be careful with high jumping and work up to it gradually. If you jump too high, you could end up with your head stuck in the ceiling or come down wrong and injure yourself.

Aerobic bouncing is the most fun of the three. It consists of jumping jacks, twisting, jogging, or sprinting in place, bouncing on one leg at a time, dancing, and any other crazy maneuvers you can think of. Put on some music you enjoy, move your body, and have fun while you get your blood pumping and your sweat on.

My typical rebounder routine is warming up for a couple of minutes with gentle health bouncing, 5 to 10 minutes alternating between strength and aerobic bouncing, and then cooling down with a couple minutes of health bouncing. I often put on headphones and listen to workout/dance music, worship music, or healing scriptures while bouncing. It's pretty hard to overdo it with rebounding, but if you feel sensitivity or pain while doing it, take it easy. While healing cancer, I did this two to three times per day.

If you are too weak to jump, some rebounders include a stabilizer bar you can hold on to, or you can simply sit on the rebounder and bounce gently in a seated position. I bought my rebounder a few months after abdominal surgery and found it too painful to jump on at first, so I started with gentle health bouncing. As my body healed, the pain went away and I was eventually able to do the strength and aerobic bouncing.

Maximize Your Rebounding Workout

➤ Do it outside. Get fresh air and sunshine and connect with God and nature (if nature permits).

➤ Take at least 10 deep breaths while bouncing. Inhale through your nose, hold it for a few seconds, and then push it out through your mouth, fully emptying your lungs.

➤ Rebound with enough intensity to break a sweat at least once per day.

Sweating is super beneficial because it helps your body detoxify specific toxins including arsenic, cadmium, lead, and mercury.[16] Saunas are an effective way to sweat out toxins, but sweaty aerobic exercise is even better because exercise turns on cancer-protective genes in your body. Either way you'll need a shower after you get sweaty. The nice thing about rebounding is that you can still get a benefit from it even if you don't break a sweat, but try to get at least one sweaty workout per day. I like to rebound first thing in the morning before I shower for the day.

SUN LOVE

Epidemiological studies suggest that we could prevent roughly 30,000 U.S. cancer deaths per year just by getting more sunshine. Regular sunlight/vitamin D intake inhibits growth of breast and colon cancer cells and is also associated with substantial decreases in death rates from these two cancers, and metabolites of vitamin D have produced complete and partial clinical responses in lymphoma patients having high vitamin D metabolite receptor levels in tumor tissue.

Severe sunburn can cause melanoma, but long-term regular sun exposure inhibits melanoma. We've been conditioned to be afraid of the sun because sun exposure can increase the risk of skin cancers that have a 0.3 percent death rate, causing about 2,000 deaths per year. But regular sun exposure prevents cancers that have death rates from 20 to 65 percent, causing 138,000 U.S. deaths per year.[17] Fifteen minutes of daily sunshine is ideal but can be difficult in winter months. Vitamin D is one of the most important anti-cancer vitamins, and I take at least 1,000 IU of vitamin D3 in supplement form every day.

RETURN TO PLANET EARTH

The most underrated form of exercise that does not require any equipment or a gym membership is walking. Walking for 10 to 20 minutes two to three times a day will do wonders for you, and grounding yourself by walking barefoot on the grass, dirt, or sand will increase the benefits even more. Walking barefoot allows your body to absorb negative ions from the surface of the earth, which have amazing benefits in your body. These negative ions act as antioxidants and have been found to improve blood flow, calm your nervous system, normalize cortisol, reduce inflammation and pain, improve immune function, and speed healing.[18]

To take the benefits of walking a step further, studies have shown that forest bathing—a fancy term for spending a few hours in the woods—increases natural killer cell activity and reduces blood pressure and stress hormones.[19,20] Some of these benefits are thought to be from breathing in phytoncides, which are aromatic compounds released into the air by trees and plants, like the compounds that make cedar smell like cedar.[21]

GET A FITNESS TRACKING GIZMO

A health-promoting gadget that may be helpful is a fitness tracker, which will show you how much exercise you're getting (or not getting) each day. It can also give key insights into the quality of your sleep. Fitness trackers are a helpful tool that will give you feedback you can use to improve your routine and incorporate more movement into your day. Most importantly, they keep you accountable and give you a sense of accomplishment when you hit your daily goals. Some folks are wary of fitness trackers because they don't like the idea of wearing an electronic device on their body 24 hours per day. However, if a fitness tracker keeps you exercising every day, I think the benefits outweigh any risks. If you are concerned about avoiding EMFs produced by fitness trackers, many newer models can be put on "airplane mode" and only sync with your phone when you tell them to. Last year someone gave me a fitness tracker as a gift. I was curious to see what kind of feedback it would give me, so I wore it for three months. It was fun seeing how many steps I took each day, how much sleep I got each night—I average 8 hours and 25 minutes—and how much my exercise routine contributed to my daily activity score. The tracker showed me exactly how much movement and exercise I need in my daily life to stay in an optimal range.

MOVEMENT IS LIFE

Depending on your situation, if you are recovering from surgery or treatment or are extremely out of shape, you may not be able to exercise much right off the bat. That's okay. Don't be discouraged. Start with light exercise like walking and gentle rebounding. Then, when you are able, try to incorporate some moderate aerobic exercise into your life like bike riding, short runs, hiking, martial arts, or fitness classes like yoga, Zumba, Jazzercise, or Pilates. Any kind of exercise that moves your body, increases your heart rate, and makes you break a sweat is wonderful. Just find something you enjoy and do it.

The latest research has shown that movement throughout the day may even more beneficial than 30 to 60 minutes of deliberate exercise once per day. There are many easy ways to incorporate more natural movement into your life, like always parking at the far end of the parking lot and taking the stairs instead of the elevator. If you sit at a desk all day, set a reminder to notify you every hour to get up, stretch your legs, and take a quick lap around the office for a few minutes. I bought myself an adjustable standing desk with a treadmill underneath, and I've never been happier with my office arrangement. The purpose of a treadmill desk is not to get a workout while you work; it's mainly just to make sure you stay in motion. Walking is better for you than standing still. Even when I set my treadmill at the slowest pace, I still manage to walk several miles per day on it. Movement is life!

NO TIME TO REST

The flip side of exercise is rest. Too much of one and not enough of the other can create an unhealthy imbalance. You need an early bedtime and lots of sleep, because sleep is when your body heals. Six to eight hours of sleep per night is considered to be the ideal range for most people, but individual needs vary. According to the CDC, more than a third of American adults aren't getting enough sleep.[22] If you're getting less than seven hours of sleep per night, you may be sleep deprived. Not getting enough sleep night after night can create a "sleep debt" that keeps growing over time and can lead to a gradual degradation of your health.

Sleep deprivation can affect your mood and brain function, including your memory, learning, creativity, and emotions. And most importantly, it can affect your physical appearance. Lack of sleep directly affects your face, causing swollen and drooping eyelids, dark circles, wrinkles, and droopy corners of your mouth. The longer you are sleep deprived, the more permanent these changes become. Sleep deprivation can also lead to depression, weight gain, a weak immune system, diabetes, heart disease, cancer, and death.

During sleep, the body produces hormones called cytokines that help fight infections. Low levels of cytokines make sleep-deprived people more susceptible to everyday infections like colds and flu. Researchers at Carnegie Mellon University found that otherwise healthy men and women who slept less than seven hours a night were three times more likely to develop cold symptoms after exposure to a cold-causing virus than people who slept eight hours or more.[23]

Before the advent of electricity, our ancestors tended to go to sleep earlier, typically within a few hours after sunset. Their sleep habits were in harmony with nature and the cycle of the sun. They slept less in the summer and more in the winter. In the winter months, they often slept for as many as twelve hours in two shifts, with one to three hours of wakefulness in the middle of the night, during which they would busy themselves reading, writing, working, praying, socializing, and, of course, getting busy.

Historical documents refer to these two sleeping shifts as first sleep and second sleep.

Electrical lighting and our modern indoor living and working environments have reduced our exposure to sunlight during the day, increased our exposure to artificial light at night, and caused our circadian clocks to be out of sync with the light-dark cycle produced by the sun. We are living in disharmony with nature.

A 2013 study found that after just one week of no exposure to artificial light, campers with varying internal biological clocks all synchronized with the light-dark cycle of the sun. Before camping their bodies began producing melatonin around 10:30 P.M., with sleep starting at 12:30 A.M. and melatonin offset happening around 8 A.M. After a week of camping, all of the campers' internal clocks shifted two hours earlier. Their bodies began producing melatonin right around sundown, with peak melatonin in the middle of the solar night and melatonin offset beginning right after sunrise.[24] Their circadian rhythms became perfectly aligned with the cycle of the sun.

Melatonin, also known as "the hormone of darkness," is produced by your pineal gland when your body detects low light in the evening. It is an antioxidant that is five times more powerful than vitamin C, and it increases the effectiveness of your lymphocytes, killer cells that fight off foreign invaders and mutated cells. In addition, melatonin increases the activity of superoxide dismutase and glutathione, which are antioxidants and detoxifiers and help repair damaged cells. Melatonin has been shown to inhibit angiogenesis and metastasis, and to promote apoptosis (cell death) in many different types of cancer cells.[25,26] The physiological surge of melatonin in your body at night is considered a "natural restraint" on tumor initiation, promotion, and progression.[27]

Exposure to artificial light, especially blue light, between dusk and bedtime can interfere with your sleep and your body's production of melatonin. Researchers found that exposure to room light (<200 lux) in the late evening reduced pre-sleep melatonin levels by 71.4 percent, shortened nighttime melatonin duration by about 90 minutes compared to dim light (<3 lux), and reduced total daily levels of melatonin by about 12.5 percent in human subjects.[28] Another study found that just 15 seconds of bright light exposure at night caused circadian disruption in participants and delayed melatonin onset by an average of 34 minutes.[29]

In the 2011 Nurses' Health Study, researchers at Harvard reported a correlation between low melatonin levels in women who worked the night shift and an increased risk of breast cancer.[30] Shorter wavelength blue light emitted by LED and fluorescent lighting, as well as electronics like TVs, smartphones, computers, some alarm clocks, and LED street lights, suppresses melatonin more than any other type of light.[31] A 2018 study found that women in urban areas exposed to high levels of outdoor blue light at night had 1.5 higher risk of breast cancer and men had a twofold increase in prostate cancer risk compared to those who were less exposed.[32] A study by the University of Toronto found that night shift workers who wore glasses that blocked blue light wavelengths produced more melatonin than those who didn't.[33] Blind women have a 35 to 50 percent lower risk of breast cancer than women who can see.[34] They tend to sleep longer and have higher levels of melatonin and lower levels of estrogen, which is reduced by melatonin.

Substances that interfere with your body's melatonin production include caffeine, tobacco, alcohol, aspirin, Ibuprofen, beta blockers, benzodiazepines, corticosteroids, and drugs that regulate serotonin like Prozac. There are over 800 brand-name and generic drugs known to interact with melatonin.[35] If you are taking any prescription drugs, they could be inhibiting your body's production of melatonin, reducing the quality of your sleep, and affecting your health. Supplementation of 20 mg of melatonin per day (before bed) along with conventional treatments has been found to cause substantial improvements in tumor remission, one-year survival, and alleviation of side effects from radiotherapy and chemotherapy.[36]

LACK OF SLEEP CAN ELEVATE YOUR CANCER RISK

A Japanese study of nearly 24,000 women ages 40 to 79 found that women who slept less than six hours a night were more likely to develop breast cancer than those who slept longer.[37] A 2010 study at Case Western Reserve University found an increased risk for colon cancer in people who slept less than six hours per night.[38]

However, just like too much exercise, too much sleep could also be unhealthy. A 2017 study found that breast cancer patients who slept more than nine hours per night had a higher risk of death than those who slept between six and eight hours. Patients who reported difficulty falling asleep or staying asleep also had increased risk of death.[39,40]

Interrupted sleep can make cancer aggressive and speed its growth. In 2014 sleep apnea researchers at the University of Chicago found that cancerous tumors in mice whose sleep was gently interrupted every two minutes grew twice as large as the tumors in the mice who had slept normally without interruption.[41] And this was after only four weeks of interrupted sleep. Before you panic, four weeks of bad sleep for a mouse is roughly the equivalent of about 2.5 years of bad sleep for a human. Practitioners of Eastern medicine claim that every hour of sleep before midnight is twice as beneficial as every hour after midnight. Whether that's true or not, 11 P.M. to 1 A.M. has been identified as a critical recharge period for many internal systems, like your adrenals.

Sleeping pills are not the answer. Taking as few as 18 sleeping pills per year triples your risk of death and taking 2 to 3 pills per week increases your risk of death by a factor of five. The risk of death from taking sleep drugs including barbiturates, benzodiazepines like Xanax and Valium, and "Z" drugs like Ambien is nearly the same as the risk with smoking.[42]

The first step to getting more sleep is setting an earlier bedtime, within a few hours after the sun goes down. Depending on your living situation, this may involve rearranging your schedule. You'll definitely need the support of the people you share a roof with. On the plus side, going to bed early usually makes it easier to get up early, which means less stress trying to get out the door in the morning. This can create time for you to read a devotional, pray, meditate, juice, work out, or plan your to-do list and meals for the day.

Exposure to bright morning light helps reset your internal clock and normalize your circadian rhythm. A 2017 study found that breast cancer patients who were exposed to bright light from a light box for 30 minutes every morning for one month had significant improvements in sleep quality and sleep time and less chronic fatigue.[43] According to one of the study authors, cancer survivors and other individuals who spend most of their days indoors may not receive enough bright light to keep their biological rhythms synchronized. Researchers recommend spending time near windows with lots of natural light and keeping the indoor lighting as bright as possible during the morning.[44]

SLEEP DETOXIFIES YOUR BRAIN

While studying the brains of sleeping mice, scientists at the University of Rochester discovered a dramatic increase in the circulation of cerebrospinal fluid going in and out of the brain. Dr. Maiken Nedergaard, professor of neurosurgery and author of the study published in *Science*, likened the process to a dishwasher, forcefully washing out all of the toxic metabolic waste that accumulated in your brain that day. The longer you stay awake, the more toxins (like beta amyloid) accumulate in your brain.[45] These toxins influence your brain chemistry and affect your ability to think clearly and rationally.

Healthy Nighttime Rituals

Here's my list of nighttime rituals to help you get the best sleep possible and optimize your body's ability to repair, regenerate, and heal.

Eat an early dinner and go to bed on an empty stomach.

Eat all your meals within an 11-hour window or less, such as 8 A.M. to 7 P.M. Researchers found that breast cancer patients who fasted less than 13 hours per night had a 36 percent higher risk for recurrence compared to those who fasted 13 hours or more.[46] Don't eat a meal before bed, and definitely do not eat in the middle of the night. Eating late at night forces your body to use energy to digest food while you sleep instead of repairing itself.

Dim the lights around your house after sundown.

This prepares your body for sleep. Take a warm bath. Use essential oils like frankincense, myrrh, and lavender to calm yourself and relax. Reading before bed can help you relax as well and get your brain and body into sleep mode. Don't turn the lights back on to brush your teeth or to use the bathroom before bed.

Avoid anything stimulating.

Caffeine, sugar, social media, and work-related activities all turn on your brain, which can make it difficult to fall asleep quickly once you get into bed. Stop watching stressful television before bed. Especially the news. Also avoid intense dramas, mysteries, horror, action/adventure shows, and sports. All of these types of entertainment excite you and raise your stress hormones, which can keep you awake and contribute to chronic stress.

Don't worry about tomorrow.

Worry will keep you awake. Don't worry about the future or tomorrow. A proven method to reduce nighttime worry and anxiety is to write down tomorrow's to-do list every night before bed. This will make you feel more organized and in control of your life, and put your mind at ease as you doze off.

Make your bedroom a cave.

Your bedroom should be cool, quiet, and dark. The ideal temperature for sound sleep is between 60 and 70 degrees Fahrenheit. If your room is much warmer or cooler, or if your blankets are too heavy or too light, you may toss and turn during the night and not get enough deep, restful sleep. It may be helpful to black out your windows or wear a sleep mask. Light at night can interfere with your body's production of melatonin, one of the most powerful anti-cancer hormones in your body.

Devices That Can Improve Sleep

Blue blockers—The nerdiest of health-nerd accessories, these orange-tinted glasses block the blue light produced by fluorescent and LED lighting and the screens of TVs and electronic devices. I often wear them at night.

Sound machine—The white noise produced by a sound machine can help you stay asleep by masking random outside noises and things that go bump in the night that might disturb your sleep. There are also sound-machine smartphone apps.

Sleep music—An alternative to a sound machine is soothing instrumental music played at specific frequencies thought to resonate with the body and promote healing.

Air purifier—Since you're in your bedroom for 7 to 10 hours every night, it makes sense to ensure you are breathing the cleanest air possible by reducing or eliminating pollutants and allergens, including pollen, pet dander, dust mites, smoke, chemical gases, bacteria, and mold. Some air purifiers have an audible fan that can serve as a sound machine.

Grounding sheet—Like walking barefoot in the grass, using a grounding sheet connects your body to the free-flowing negative ions on the surface of the earth. I use a grounding pad under my keyboard while working at my desk, and I sleep on a grounding sheet as well.

Sunrise alarm clock—Unlike jarring buzzers or a blaring radio that shock you out of deep sleep, a sunrise alarm clock wakes you naturally by gradually filling the room with light over the course of several minutes.

Organic mattress—Most commercial mattresses are made with synthetic fibers and treated with toxic flame retardants, which can off-gas chemical fumes that you breathe in all night. An organic mattress is a big investment that may require saving up for, but it's worth it. We sleep on an organic latex foam mattress.

Sleep mask and ear plugs—If you can't get your room dark enough, or if you travel a lot, you might benefit from wearing ear plugs and/or a sleep mask over your eyes.

For an updated list of the products I use in my bedroom to optimize my sleep, go to www.chrisbeatcancer.com/sleep.

A DAY OF REST

The final component in rest is setting aside an entire day for it every week. A day of rest may seem strange in our culture obsessed with productivity and achievement, but this is a biblical principle dating back to Genesis, and it's even one of the Ten Commandments.

Remember the sabbath day, to keep it holy. Six days you shall labor and do all your work, but the seventh day is a sabbath of the LORD your God; in it you shall not do any work, you or your son or your daughter, your male or your female servant or your cattle or your sojourner who stays with you. For in six days the LORD made the heavens and the earth, the sea and all that is in them, and rested on the seventh day; therefore the LORD blessed the sabbath day and made it holy. (Exodus 20:8–11) (NASB)

In Japan's competitive corporate culture, employees routinely work 60 to 100 hours per week, in some cases not taking days off for months. It's become such a problem that they even have a word for one of its tragic consequences: *karoshi*, which means death from overwork. The stress induced by working too much has been found to cause heart attacks and strokes as well as depression-related suicide.

So what does a day of rest look like? It is one day per week where you don't do physical or mental work and you don't require people to work for you. On our day of rest, we go to church, sometimes have lunch with friends or family, and then usually take naps and relax for the rest of the day. We might read, watch a movie, play a game with the kids, or have dinner with in-laws, but that's about it.

Doing nothing may be hard for you if you enjoy working or feel pressure to be productive, but your body and brain need a break. Don't think about work. Don't talk about work. Don't check your e-mail. Stay off the internet if it's work related. And just try to be at peace. The less physical energy you exert on your day of rest, the more benefit you will receive from it. Making yourself take a day of rest is important not only to maintain your health, but to restore it.

Massive Action Steps for Exercise and Rest

➤ Commit to 30 to 60 minutes of aerobic exercise per day six days per week (walking counts).

➤ Exercise outside in the fresh air and sunshine as much as possible.

➤ Get sweaty at least once per day six days per week.

➤ Get a few minutes of sunshine on your body every day.

➤ Walk barefoot in the grass for a few minutes every day.

➤ Spend a few hours in nature "forest bathing" at least once per week.

➤ Park farther away than you normally would and take the stairs instead of the elevator.

➤ Stand up every hour or so, take a walk around the office, and move your body.

➤ Consider investing in a treadmill desk.

➤ Eat your meals in an 11-hour window.

➤ Go to bed within a few hours of sundown.

➤ Make your bedroom cool, quiet, and dark.

➤ Consider investing in tools and devices to improve your exercise habits and sleep.

➤ Take one day of rest every week.

UNDER PRESSURE

Stress and Negative Emotions

Worry is a misuse of the imagination.

— DAN ZADRA

Worry never robs tomorrow of its sorrow. It only saps today of its joy.

— LEO BUSCAGLIA

WHEN I GRADUATED FROM COLLEGE, the countdown to marriage began. My wedding date was only six months away and I needed to get my act together. So, as I mentioned earlier, I took a job at a financial firm. It wasn't what I had planned on, but I had sales experience and a business degree, and the man who recruited me made it sound pretty lucrative. I started out in financial planning selling life insurance and annuities, with eventual plans to become a fully licensed investment broker. There was no salary. It was straight commission with a small weekly draw, and I was constantly stressed about finding new clients and whether I was going to make enough money to keep the job.

The following year I started buying rental properties and had to learn how to get houses renovated and rented, and how to manage tenants. I was having loads more fun investing in real estate than I ever did in the insurance business, but I was still stressed. I was working longer and harder than I had ever worked in my life. I was burning the candle at both ends, living on adrenaline, sugar, caffeine, and fast food, and I was not taking care of myself. The year after that, the abdominal pains started. Then in December came the cancer diagnosis.

Stress can make you sick. And kill you.

I've counseled a lot of people with cancer over the years, and the one thing they all have in common is stress. The human body is intelligently designed with a survival mechanism triggered by anything your mind perceives as threatening. This is known as a fight-or-flight response. Any time you find yourself in a thrilling, dangerous, or life-threatening situation, like riding a roller coaster, watching a scary movie, or looking down the barrel of a gun, your body automatically kicks into survival mode.

If you are confronted by a tiger, the first thing that happens is a sense: danger. Followed by a thought: *I'm about to be tiger food.* That thought triggers an emotion: fear. That emotion triggers the release of stress hormones (adrenaline and cortisol), which activate a physical response in your body. Simply put, these hormones divert all of your available energy to your muscles and the parts of your brain that can assist you in survival. Adrenaline gives you strength and power. Cortisol tells your body to dump glucose into your bloodstream, making you more alert and giving you a burst of energy to run faster and farther, or fight harder.

If a tiger came after you and you somehow managed to escape, your body would eventually shift out of fight-or-flight mode and back to normal operation. Once the stressful event is over, the stress hormones stop pumping, the fear subsides, your mind and body relax, and all of your other bodily functions that have been "paused," like digestion and immune function, come back online.

Have you ever been so upset that you can't think straight? Or sat down to take a test and your memory was blank? Or heard someone say they couldn't remember what happened after a traumatic event? Stress hormones did that. The reason stress hormones switch off your immune system, digestive system, reproductive system, and parts of your brain is simple: energy conservation. Your brain uses about 20 percent of your energy. Your digestive system uses about 15 percent of your energy—sometimes more, which is why eating a heavy meal can make you sleepy. Your body is brilliantly designed to direct energy to where it is needed most. In a true fight-or-flight situation, that would be your muscles.

The hormones produced by stress are a very good thing in the proper context and can help save your life. In a real fight-or-flight situation, they can help you escape from a swarm of bad guys, hightail it out of there, or even lift a car off someone trapped underneath, Superman style. That kind of stress is called acute stress—a short-term stressful situation with a beginning and an end. But acute stress events are few and far between, and very rare for most of us in first-world nations. Our problem is something very different. Our problem is chronic stress.

THE TIGER YOU CAN'T ESCAPE

Chronic stress is the grinding, day in, day out stress caused by the worries, fears, responsibilities, and conflicts we have in life. It is like the tiger that you can never get away from. It's always behind you—stalking you. You have to keep moving. And you can't rest for long. You are running from it every day, from the time you wake up until the time you go to sleep, and sometimes it even wakes you up in the middle of the night.

We are stressed to the max in our modern world, and stressors are coming at us from all sides: negative and dramatic media, financial difficulties, family demands and problems, toxic relationships, social pressures, work demands, bad lifestyle habits like self-abuse, lack of sleep, stimulants, and even too much exercise.

Stress starts in the mind and manifests in the body. Chronic stress produces elevated levels of adrenaline and cortisol, which keep you in a constant state of "flight-or-flight light" and can lead to all sorts of problems over time, like chronic fatigue from exhaustive depletion (adrenal failure); depression; nervousness; hypertension; a reduction in your body's ability to digest and absorb the nutrients in food; digestive problems like ulcers, Crohn's disease, and colitis; hormone problems; a decrease in male testosterone and sperm count; irregular menstrual cycles and fertility problems in women; and mostly importantly, immune suppression, which increases the likelihood of developing a chronic disease in the body, like cancer. Simply put, when stress hormones are up, your immune system is down.

Cortisol causes a release of sugar into your bloodstream for energy, but later causes intense sugar cravings to replenish glucose reserves. This leads to impulsive and irrational stress eating, which almost always involves extremely unhealthy, high-sugar "comfort foods" like pizza, pasta, ice cream, candy, snack foods, and sugary drinks. Prolonged elevated blood glucose promotes inflammation and fuels cancer growth if it is not used by muscle activity.

Stress also interferes with your brain function. When you are under stress, parts of your brain are switched off—affecting your ability to think rationally—and your lower brain stem (aka your reptilian brain) becomes dominant. The reptilian brain controls your instinctive survival responses like anger, aggressive dominant behavior, fear, revenge, tribalism, territorial behavior, and reproductive impulses. The reptilian brain is primitive, impulsive, and irrational, which is why people who are in a state of fear, worry, anxiety, anger, or sexual arousal often make impulsive, irrational, and really bad decisions. Extreme rage can make you temporarily insane.

In 2013 researchers reported that anti-cancer drugs didn't work as well in mice under stress because adrenaline turns off the mechanism that tells cancer cells to die. The mice were then given a beta blocker to block adrenaline production, which slowed down their heart rate, lowered their blood pressure, and restored their immune function. When adrenaline production was inhibited, the mice did not have accelerated tumor growth even when put under stress.[1] Another study found that mice put under stress had six times the spread of cancer.[2] According to study author and cancer biologist Dr. Erica Sloan, "Stress sends a signal into the cancer that allows tumor cells to escape from the cancer and spread through the body."[3]

Stress has the same effect on cancer in humans. Stress activates a gene in immune system cells called ATF3 that causes them to malfunction and help cancer cells spread throughout the body. Both breast cancer patients and mice with activated ATF3 in their immune cells were found to have lower survival rates than those without activated ATF3. This cancer-promoting stress gene can also be turned on by chemotherapy, radiation, and poor diet.[4]

Without exception, every single cancer patient I've met had major chronic stress in their life besides cancer. And in many cases, it wasn't just one thing. It was a combination of several significant stressors persisting in their life for many years. Many of us are teetering on the brink of disease. Then a major stressful event happens, which is the cancer trigger, the tipping point that pushes us over the edge. The death or disability of a loved one, betrayal, a divorce or bad breakup, the loss of a job, insults, injuries, and harassment. Even moving, marriage, and pregnancy fall into this category. Many patients I've talked to are able to pinpoint one or more traumatic cancer-trigger events that happened to them in the five years before their diagnosis. And of course, a cancer diagnosis only makes matters worse. A cancer diagnosis or recurrence is a stress bomb. The fear and worry that accompany a diagnosis can be profoundly immunosuppressant and a catalyst for accelerated cancer growth and metastasis in the body. This is why it is critical to identify and eliminate all the stresses in your life.

STRESS. OUT.

The first step in reducing stress is to stop worrying. Worrying is a bad habit that you can break. Stop worrying about your health, about other people, about the economy, about the government, about the future, and about events you cannot control. To worry is to live in fear.

As a Christian, I looked to the Bible for answers. The words of Jesus, Paul, and Peter gave me clarity and peace and showed me how to overcome fear, anxiety, and worry.

Jesus said, "Do not worry about your life, what you will eat or drink; or about your body, what you will wear . . . But seek first his kingdom and his righteousness, and all these things will be given to you as well. Therefore, do not worry about tomorrow, for tomorrow will worry about itself. Each day has enough trouble of its own." (Matthew 6:25–34) (NIV)

Paul said, "Don't worry about anything; instead, pray about everything. Tell God what you need, and thank him for all he has done. Then you will experience God's peace, which exceeds anything we can understand." (Philippians 4:6–7) (NIV)

Peter said, ". . . Humble yourselves under the mighty hand of God, that He may exalt you at the proper time, casting all your anxiety on Him, because He cares for you." (1 Peter 5:6–7) (NASB)

Worry and doubt are the opposite of faith. I realized that exercising my faith meant trusting God to lead me, to protect me, to provide for me and my family, and to heal me. Fully trusting Him meant letting go of my fear, choosing to believe and not to doubt.

As part of my daily routine, every time I felt worried and afraid, this is what I prayed:

> Lord, I am not going to be afraid. I am giving you my fear. Jesus, I am laying it at your feet. I trust you with my life, my health, my family, my finances, my future. I trust you. Thank you for leading me in the path of healing, for supplying all my needs, and for working everything out for my good. Amen.

THE LIFE-CHANGING MAGIC OF PROBLEM SOLVING

Marie Kondo wrote an international best-seller on how to get rid of clutter in your home called *The Life-Changing Magic of Tidying Up*. If you are one of the few people left on the planet who haven't read it, the premise is simple. One by one, go through every item you own and ask yourself whether or not it brings you joy. If it doesn't bring you joy, throw it out. The power of this method is that it requires you to systematically evaluate everything you own. In the same way, you need to focus your attention on identifying and dealing with the stress-producing problems in your life that you've been avoiding.

Many of the problems we have in life persist unnecessarily simply because we put off solving them. We avoid them, ignore them, procrastinate, and in some cases even deny they exist. Some problems and stressors in life resolve on their own, but others will not go away until you take action. Everyone has problems in their life that they need to solve. Now is the time to face your problems head-on, take Massive Action, and get busy solving them. And as you do, you will feel the weight of stress and anxiety lifted off you.

Make a two-column list with Problems on one side and Solutions on the other. In the left-hand column, list your problems and sources of stress. Ask yourself, *What am I worried about? What is causing me the most stress? Who is causing me the most stress?* Once that is done, review each stress-producer in your life and then ask yourself, *What do I need to do to remove this stress from my life?* Write your answer on the right-hand side of the list. This practice engages the creative problem-solving part of your brain. Most problems have a simple solution—not necessarily an easy solution, but a simple one. For example, if your problem is bitterness toward an ex, the solution is that you need to forgive. If your problem is that you are in an abusive relationship, the solution is that you need to leave and get help, and you need to forgive.

Identify the largest sources of stress on the list and tackle those first. Dealing with the big problems will give you the biggest bang for your buck in terms of stress reduction. Chronic stress will not only make you sick, but it will keep you sick. That's why it's imperative that you eliminate as many sources of stress and negativity from your life as quickly as possible. If friends or family members are stressing you out, tell them you need space or distance yourself from them for the time being. If you are trying to heal cancer or another chronic disease, this is a time to be a little selfish. It's okay. You have to take care of yourself first if you want to be around to take care of others. Finally, some of your problems are out of your control and cannot be solved by you. Those are the ones you give to God.

Massive Action Steps for Stress Reduction

➤ Identify the sources of stress in your life.

➤ Make a to-do list to eliminate every stress in your life.

➤ Get busy removing stresses and solving your problems.

➤ Stop worrying. Give your fears and worries to God daily and trust Him to take care of you.

➤ Read *How to Stop Worrying and Start Living* by Dale Carnegie.

➤ Laugh! One hour of stand-up comedy can boost your immune system for up to 12 hours.[5]

➤ Sing! Singing for an hour reduces stress hormones and boosts your immune system.[6]

SPIRITUAL HEALING

Do not be wise in your own eyes.
Fear the LORD and turn away from evil.
It will be healing to your body and refreshment to your bones.

— PROVERBS 3:7-8 (NASB)

CANCER FORCED ME to step out in faith and trust God in a way that I never had before. I had never had a crisis like this in my life. I had never known this kind of desperation. I had never felt like my life was completely out of my control. Cancer threatened to cut my life short, and I knew I needed help from above. My faith and my relationship with God were a huge part of my healing journey.

I grew up in a Christian home. I came to know Jesus at a young age, but as I got older I saw some things in the church I didn't like, and I used that as an excuse to rebel. I gravitated toward other rebellious kids who were not good influences, and by the time I was 16, my relationship with God was practically nonexistent. When I was 21, in the midst of working, going to college, and seeing an emptiness in what the world had to offer, I decided to make my relationship with God a priority in my life. I got plugged into a local church and began attending Bible studies, going on church retreats, and growing in my faith. Five years later the colon cancer diagnosis happened. Micah and I had just celebrated our two-year anniversary and I was playing on the church worship team every Sunday. In the midst of the shock, fear, anxiety, confusion, frustration, and everything else that comes with a cancer diagnosis, I remembered Romans 8:28 (NIV):

And we know that God works all things for the good of those who love Him, who have been called according to His purpose.

Cancer was not good news. I did not see it as a gift or a blessing. It was the worst thing that had ever happened to me. But I chose to believe that God was going to work this bad thing out for my good. In my fear I made the choice to believe and I said, "Okay, God, I don't understand why this is happening, but I'm going to believe that You are going to work this for my good."

As I read through the Bible looking for encouragement, I came across Psalm 34. The Sunday after I was diagnosed, my wife and I stood up in front of our church and I made the dreaded announcement. "Hi, everybody. I've been diagnosed with colon cancer . . . but I'm choosing to believe this promise in Psalm 34:19 (NIV):

The righteous person may have many troubles, but the LORD delivers him from them all.

And I said, "This is my verse. God is going to deliver me from this."

After surgery I prayed and said, "God, if there's another way besides chemo, please show me . . ." Two days later I received the book *God's Way to Ultimate Health*, which helped me understand that it didn't make sense to pray and ask for healing while continuing to do the things that could be making me sick. I knew I needed to take Massive Action to change my life and rebuild my body as part of the process, and I believed that in doing so I would be delivered from my affliction.

There's a beautiful story in the Bible about a woman who came to Jesus for healing. She had what was described as "an issue of blood." She had a bleeding condition. And because of this, according to Jewish religious law, she was considered unclean and untouchable and had lived as an outcast from her own people for 12 years. And it said, "She had suffered a great deal under the care of many doctors and had spent all she had, yet instead of getting better she grew worse." (Mark 5:6) (NIV)

After hearing about Jesus, she came up in the crowd behind Him and touched His cloak, and immediately her bleeding stopped. Jesus, perceiving that power had gone out of Him, turned around in the crowd and said, "Who touched my garments?" And his disciples said, "The crowd is pressing in on you and you're asking who touched you?" Jesus looked around and saw the woman, and He knew that she was the one who had touched Him. She fell down trembling before Him and told him that she was sick and that she had come to touch His garment. And Jesus said to her, "Daughter, your faith has made you well. Go in peace and be healed of your affliction." (Matthew 9:18, Mark 5:24, Luke 8:41) (NASB)

I met a woman at a conference a few years ago who came up to me and said, "I was diagnosed with cancer. And in my prayer life, I became just like that woman who needed a touch from Jesus, and God healed me." She had experienced miraculous healing and her cancer was gone. I could barely keep it together as she told me her story—because I knew where she had been. I'd been there too—down on my knees, desperate for a touch from God. Yes, I radically changed my whole life. I took responsibility for my health, for my diet and lifestyle, and for my environment, but at the end of the day, I was depending on God to lead me and to heal me.

THE POWER OF I AM

Your thoughts and beliefs create your reality and shape your future. As you think, so you are. Even though this concept has been rebranded many times as the Power of Positive Thinking, the Law of Attraction, and the Secret, and may seem a bit cliché, it is timeless truth.

Your thoughts, beliefs, and expectations are much more powerful than you realize. Regardless of the type of treatment, patients who believe a therapy is going to work have a higher likelihood of getting well and are often the ones who defy the odds, while patients who don't believe a therapy is going to help them tend to do worse. Something incredible happens when you start thinking positively and seeing yourself in a way that you may not yet be. The process starts in your mind and translates into your body. Early in my healing journey I realized that I had nothing to lose, so I changed the way I thought and I started thinking of myself as I wanted to be: healed, healthy, and well.

The placebo effect is a pervasive medically documented phenomenon. Studies in both laboratory and clinical settings consistently show that when people ingest a pharmacologically inert substance (a placebo) but believe that it is an active substance, they experience both the subjective sensations and physiologic effects expected from that active substance.[1]

In nearly every drug trial, some patients who are given a sugar pill instead of the real medication get the same benefit because they believed they would. There are also numerous documented cases of patients who got better after a fake surgery that they thought was real. A systematic review of 53 placebo-controlled surgeries found that in 51 percent of the trials, the measurable benefit in the fake surgery group was the exact same as the surgery group! The other 49 percent of placebo surgery trials reported that real surgery was more beneficial than fake surgery, but only generally by a small margin.[2]

The flip side of the placebo effect is called the nocebo effect. Some patients who expect a medication or treatment to cause them harm or have negative side effects, even if they are taking a placebo, end up experiencing those negative side effects. As a result of these phenomena, some patients who believe that chemotherapy will cure them are cured by the placebo effect. And others who believe chemo will not cure them and will cause them more harm may be amplifying its harmful effects. Your attitude, expectations, and beliefs can be more powerful than drugs or surgery. That's why it's so important to choose to think positively.

Positive thinking and affirmations may remind you of Al Franken's *Saturday Night Live* skits from the '90s, where Stuart Smalley looks at himself in the mirror and says, "I'm good enough. I'm smart enough. And doggone it, people like me." As silly as this may seem, don't discount affirmations. They can be a transformative, life-changing practice. You will be amazed at how good you feel when you make it a daily practice to encourage yourself, think positively, and see yourself as well.

No one talks to you more than *you*. Instead of depending on encouragement from others, which you may or may not get, start encouraging yourself. You can apply this to every area of your life. "I am smart. I am strong. I am courageous. I am loved. I am worthy of love. I am blessed. I am attractive. I am successful. I belong here. I am valuable. I am healed. I am healthy. I am well. And doggone it, people like me!" Stop criticizing yourself and encourage yourself instead. And talk to your body. Talk to your organs. Tell them to be healed and to be well. Choose to love yourself.

One of the most famous healing scriptures in the Bible is Isaiah 53:5 (NKJV), where the prophet Isaiah, predicting Jesus the Messiah, says "He was wounded for our transgressions. He was bruised for our iniquities. The chastisement for our peace was upon Him. And by His stripes we are healed."

Every day throughout the day, I would meditate on this verse and pray it out loud over my body, over and over again. I would say, "By Your stripes I am healed, I am healthy, and I am well, in the name of Jesus." I was exercising my faith and trusting in the redeeming work that Jesus did on the cross, and I was speaking life and health into my body.

DEALING WITH DOUBT

In John 14 (NASB) Jesus says, "Whatever you ask in My name, I will do, that the Father may be glorified in the Son. If you ask Me anything in My name, I will do it." And that's why when I prayed and asked for healing, I did it in the name of Jesus.

"Father, I'm asking for healing in the name of Jesus. And I'm believing You're going to do it, because You said that whatever I ask in Your Name You will do. I'm holding You to Your word. And I'm choosing to believe that, and that only. And I'm not going to doubt it."

Doubt can creep in, but doubt is just a thought, and you can change your thoughts. Faith is a choice. It is a practice and a discipline. Every person needs to work on this, and I still work on it daily. When doubts creep in, I just say to myself, *No, I'm not going to doubt. I'm going to believe.*

When I was struggling with fear and doubt, I often put worship music on in my headphones or in my car, sang along, got choked up, and let the emotions flow. What I found in my spiritual journey was that the very act of worship, of focusing my attention on God and not on my problems, encouraged me, strengthened my faith, and became an antidote for fear and doubt.

FAITH VERSUS FEAR

As a culture we have been conditioned to put our faith, hope, and trust in doctors first. But I want to encourage you to put your faith, hope, and trust in God first.

You need to make faith-based decisions, not fear-based decisions.

Don't let anyone use fear to motivate you, because fear-based decisions are often irrational, emotional, and unwise decisions. And fear-based decisions are often the wrong ones.

A powerful thing to ask God in prayer besides "Show me what I need to do" is "Show me what I need to change." If you ask God to show you what you need to change in your life, He will. Things will come to mind that you know are wrong and that you need to address. Ask and listen. Then take action and make those changes.

WHY ME?

A question a lot of cancer patients ask, especially if they are people of faith, is "Why did God allow this to happen?"

At the time of my diagnosis, I couldn't help but think, *This is so unfair. There are thieves and rapists and murderers . . . evil people doing evil things every day. They deserve cancer! I don't deserve cancer. I'm one of the good guys! I'm playing music in church every Sunday morning, for Pete's sake! I'm not lying, cheating, and stealing from people. I've tried to put God first in my life for the last five years and now I've got cancer? Come on!*

I know "life isn't fair," but cancer at 26 felt especially unfair. Throughout my life I had heard people say, "Whatever happens is God's will." If they were right, then that meant God wanted me to have cancer, a proposition that I didn't like and that didn't line up with the God I knew. So rather than accept that belief, I decided to study the scriptures to find out for myself whether it was God's will for me to be sick, or whether it was His will for me to be well. And what I found ignited my faith and restored my hope that I would be healed.

Psalm 103 (NIV) says, "Praise the LORD, my soul and forget not all His benefits, who forgives all your sins and heals all your diseases, who redeems your life from the pit, and crowns you with love and compassion, who satisfies your desires with good things, so that your youth is renewed like the eagle's."

I found promises of health and healing throughout the Bible. When I looked at the life and ministry of Jesus with fresh eyes, I realized that Jesus wasn't just a teacher. Jesus was a healer.

Jesus spent most of his time with the poor and the outcasts of society, the people no one cared about. He taught them about the Kingdom of God and about right and wrong, and showed them love by His actions. He performed miracles and He healed the sick over, and over, and over again. Jesus demonstrated God's great love for us in the way He served the needy and by taking the punishment for our sins on the cross. Here are just a few of the many accounts of Jesus healing the sick, documented in the book of Matthew, that ignited my faith.

"When evening came, they brought to Him many who were demon-possessed, and He cast out the spirits with a word, and healed all who were ill." (Matthew 8:16) (NASB)

In Matthew, Chapter 12, Jesus says to a man with a crippled hand, "Stretch out your hand." The man stretched it out and it was restored to normal, like his other hand. After that, the religious leaders conspired against Jesus on how to destroy Him. Jesus was aware of this, so he left. And many people followed Him, and He healed them all, and warned them not to tell who He was. (Matthew 12:9–16) (NASB)

"When Jesus went ashore, He saw a large crowd and felt compassion for them and healed their sick." (Matthew 14:14) (NASB)

"Large crowds came to Jesus, bringing with them those who were lame, crippled, blind, mute, and many others, and they laid them down at his feet; and He healed them." (Matthew 15:30) (NASB)

HEALING YOUR HEART

Bitterness, resentment, and unforgiveness are three of the most destructive emotional states, and they will rot you from the inside out and destroy your health. Now is the time to exercise your forgiveness muscle and forgive everyone who has ever hurt you.

Get into a quiet, prayerful state and close your eyes. Next search your memory for all the people who have hurt you. Think through your life chronologically. Go back as far you can—all the way back to your childhood. Family members, friends, schoolmates, strangers, co-workers . . .

Even seemingly insignificant events from your childhood may have caused deep emotional wounds that need to be healed. If you can still remember the offense, there's a chance it may still be affecting you today. If the memory triggers an emotion, that's a signal that there may be some forgiveness that needs to happen.

Take time to remember every single person who has hurt you and forgive each and every one of them, by name.

Revisiting all the times you've been hurt is something most people don't do and don't want to do. I know it's hard. But this is a critical step. Do not skip this part of the healing process. The thing you want to do least is usually the thing you need to do most. Bitterness can be a barrier to healing. You can radically change your diet and lifestyle and do all the therapies in the world, but if you don't forgive the people who have hurt you and let go of your anger and bitterness toward them, you may not get well.

When you let go of the past and choose to forgive, God will heal your heart and change you. When you pray to forgive, don't just think it. Say it out loud. Speak it out of your mouth. It's powerful. As you are thinking of each person who hurt you, pray this way:

> God. You know what they did. And you know how I feel about it. They hurt me . . . but today, right now, I'm choosing to forgive them. I am letting them go. And I am giving them to you. I am not going to carry this anger and bitterness anymore. I am laying it at your feet. It's all yours. Thank you for forgiving me, and for healing my heart and healing my body. And I'm asking you to have mercy on them and to bless them, in Jesus' name. Amen.

Love them? Bless them? Pray for them? Believe me, that's the last thing I want to do for someone who has hurt me. When someone wrongs me, I want justice, vengeance—that's human nature. But remember: we reap what we sow. When you plant a seed in the ground, you don't grow another seed; you harvest a plant with hundreds or thousands of seeds. People who sow bad seeds in life will reap an exponential harvest of bad things on themselves, much more than they sowed.

I find tremendous comfort in knowing that people will eventually get what they deserve. That makes it easier to let the offenses go. And in the meantime, I just follow Jesus' instructions and ask God to have mercy on the people who have hurt me and to bless them. Jesus emphasized the importance of forgiveness throughout his ministry. When He taught his disciples how to pray, he instructed them to pray, "Forgive us our sins as we forgive those who sin against us." It doesn't matter if you don't feel like it or if you don't feel sincere when you pray to forgive someone. Just keep on forgiving.

FORGIVENESS IS NOT A FEELING

Forgiveness is a decision. You choose to forgive despite your feelings. *I'll forgive them when they're sorry and when they apologize.* Nope. That's not going to work. Because some people will never be sorry and never apologize. The act of forgiveness is not for them; it is for you.

Forgiveness is not a one-shot deal. It is a choice for life. It is choosing to no longer hold what someone did against them. Forgiveness is choosing to show them love by letting it go, forever. If you decided to eat healthy for one week and then went back to junk food, how much would it benefit you? Forgiveness works the same way. It only works if you stick with it.

Some memories may still cause you grief and pain after you've made the decision to forgive. If that happens, you must remind yourself that you made a decision to forgive and that you're sticking with your decision. Don't let those old hurts and emotions get a foothold in your mind. Continue giving them back to God, and I assure you there will come a point in time when the forgiveness will be complete in your heart. You will see them in a new way and the pain will be gone. Going forward, make a decision to forgive new offenses quickly.

ASKING OTHERS FOR FORGIVENESS

The next part of the process is asking for forgiveness from the people that you have hurt. This is an okay place to play your cancer card if you have one. A conversation could go something like this:

"Hey, John. It's Chris . . . I don't know if you've heard, but I was diagnosed with cancer recently . . . It's made me realize that I need make some things right . . . I'm calling to ask you to forgive me for [insert offense here]. What I did was wrong and I am truly sorry. I also wanted to ask if there was anything I can do to make it up to you . . ."

Some people may graciously forgive you and others may not. They may even unleash a verbal assault on you that they think you deserve. And maybe you do deserve it. If the latter happens, don't defend yourself, don't argue, and definitely don't try to justify your actions or tell them that they were wrong too. Just let them say what they need to say. The most important thing is that you humble yourself, admit you were wrong, ask for forgiveness, and exit the conversation gracefully. This can be a powerful first step to mending a broken relationship.

GOD IS WILLING TO FORGIVE YOU

Guilt and shame about mistakes you've made in the past can lead to depression and self-hatred, which will make you miserable and sick. If you've cheated people, stolen from them, betrayed their trust, used them, and hurt them, you can push those memories aside and forget about them for a while, but ultimately you can never get away from them. Unresolved spiritual and emotional issues stay in your subconscious, raising your overall anxiety and unhappiness, and often lead to self-medication and destructive behaviors.

When you are born, your heart is pure and innocent, like a glass of purified water. One sin, the first lie you ever told, is like a tiny drop of sewage in the glass. One drop renders the water impure—polluted and undrinkable. Now imagine every bad thing you've thought or done in your life as another drop of sewage in that glass, or, to put it another way, as a black spot on your heart. We've all done shameful things that have polluted and corrupted our hearts, and we all need forgiveness.

Sin separates us from God, but Jesus Christ took the punishment for our sins on the cross, making a bridge between us and God. When God forgives you, He wipes the slate clean. Your hardened, black heart is transplanted with a new heart. And the most beautiful thing of all is that you simply have to turn to Him and ask. He loves you so much and is willing to forgive you and will not hold your past mistakes against you. Knowing that God loves you and is quick to forgive makes it possible to forgive yourself and let go of the guilt and shame you've been carrying.

One of the last things Jesus said when he was dying on the cross, innocent of any wrongdoing, was "Father forgive them, for they know not what they do."

If Jesus was able to forgive those who conspired against Him and those who beat Him, whipped Him, spit on Him, nailed Him to a cross, and mocked Him while He was dying, you can forgive the people in your life who have hurt you.

In my search for answers, all the roads I ventured down brought me to the same place. Whether God struck me with cancer or it was the result of my choices or the choices of others became irrelevant, and I realized that I had only one appropriate response—to surrender. Once I made that act of surrender, it opened the door to some of the sweetest and most powerful times in my life. He gave me peace in the middle of the storm, and He carried me through to the other side. I don't view cancer as a gift or a blessing, but God worked it for my good and used it to bless my life.

JUST ASK

If you don't know God, if you don't know if there is a God, all you have to do is reach out and ask. Just get alone, get quiet, and say, "Okay, God, here I am. I'm ready. I'm open. I'm willing to believe. Just reveal Yourself to me. I want to know You." I'm certain that if you continue to pray that way, God will reveal Himself to you and He will speak to you. Amazing, incredible, supernatural things will happen in your life. You just have to humble yourself and ask.

"Ask and it will be given to you; seek and you will find; knock and the door will be opened to you."
— MATTHEW 7:7 (NIV)

Finally, find a Bible and read about the life and the words of Jesus. Read the books of Matthew, Mark, Luke, and John. If you want to know God's heart, you'll see it in Jesus.

Massive Action Steps to Spiritual Healing

➤ Choose faith over fear and doubt.

➤ Give your fears, worries, and anxiety to God and trust Him to lead you.

➤ Catch yourself when you are thinking negatively and choose to think positively.

➤ Always look for the silver lining in every situation.

➤ Encourage yourself every day.

➤ Visualize yourself being well.

➤ Speak life and health into your body.

➤ Forgive everyone who has ever hurt you.

➤ Ask for forgiveness from those you have hurt.

➤ Be quick to forgive going forward.

➤ Get right with God. Surrender. Reach out and ask for forgiveness, help, and healing.

➤ Ask God to show you what you need to do and what you need to change.

➤ Find a Bible and read Matthew, Mark, Luke, and John.

EPILOGUE

LIFE IS A JOURNEY full of obstacles, roadblocks, detours, and miracles. Sometimes you find yourself traveling with companions, and sometimes your journey separates you from the people you care about and you have to travel alone. Sometimes your paths intersect again down the road. Sometimes they don't. Sometimes you realize you're going the wrong way and you have to turn around and retrace your steps. Sometimes you have to completely abandon your path and start a new one.

In his poem "The Road Not Taken," Robert Frost reflects on his choice to take the road less traveled and how it "made all the difference." In my Robert Frost moment, the popular path—the conventional road—was enticing. It was easy.

Conventional cancer treatment required nothing from me except to show up. It was a permission slip to not change, to keep living the life that was killing me. Chemo put God in a box. He was either going to cure me with chemo or He wasn't—it was not up to me. I was tempted to get on the conventional train, relinquish control of my life, and be a passenger. It appealed to my reluctance to examine my life, to face my faults and my flaws, and to admit my mistakes. It appealed to my narcissism that I was just unlucky, a victim, and that nothing that happened to me was ever my fault. That's not to say conventional treatment or chemotherapy is wrong for everyone, but those are the reasons it was wrong for me.

The alternate path—the road less traveled—was hard. And it was lonely. I had no idea where it would take me, and I knew it would be challenging, but I sensed it would make me stronger and wiser. Deep in my core, it made the most sense. Despite the opinions of many people around me, I knew this was the path I had to take. I didn't like who I was, and I didn't want to change. But I knew I had to change to survive. I embraced the fear of failure, the fear of the unknown, the fear of death, and the adventure of it all. I savored the thrill of being alive and the freedom to live or die on my own terms. And I felt powerful. Once I made the decision to step out in faith, into the unknown, I had peace. And I knew that if I made it through the jungle, I could show others the way.

Maybe you are at the same crossroad. Fighting doubt and fear. Trying to decide what to do next and frustrated because there are no good options, no guarantees. Maybe your instincts are telling you to do the opposite of everyone else, but maybe you are afraid of criticism and rejection. Maybe you are afraid of failure. Maybe you've been telling yourself you aren't worthy of health or success or happiness. You are. Now is the time to start telling yourself that you are. Now is the time to stop criticizing yourself and start encouraging yourself. Your thoughts and actions create your reality and your future. Changing your thoughts and actions can change the course of your life.

This is your journey. You are the navigator. You are the author of your story. Don't let anyone rush you into things you don't understand. Don't do anything that doesn't make sense to you. Don't let anyone take the wheel from you. Don't let anyone manipulate you with fear. Make decisions that are based on facts and faith, not fear. Listen to your instincts and intuition. Listen to your gut. Listen to the Holy Spirit. Pray. Reach out. Ask God for help. Ask for signs. Ask for direction. Ask God to show you what you need to do, and what you need to change. Both faith and doubt are a choice. Choose faith. Be strong and courageous.

You may be afraid, but courage cannot exist without fear. Courage is the decision to move forward in spite of fear. Fear is the darkness that courage shines through. Now is the time to start your healing adventure. It just takes one step . . .

May you prosper in good health even as your soul prospers.

RESOURCES

THE END OF THIS BOOK is just the beginning. I have so much more to share with you! For bonus content and resources, including my free patient guide *20 Questions for Your Oncologist*, interviews with holistic survivors, access to our community of thrivers, helpful links, and more, please visit

www.chrisbeatcancer.com/bookresources

ENDNOTES

CHAPTER 1: Into the Jungle

1. University of Chicago Medicine, "Evidence Mounts for Link Between Opioids and Cancer Growth," *UChicago Medicine* (Mar 2012). http://www .uchospitals.edu/news/2012/20120321-opioid.html (accessed Apr 2018).

2. Jay Soong-Jin Lee et al, "New Persistent Opioid Use Among Patients with Cancer After Curative-Intent Surgery," *Journal of Clinical Oncology* 35.36 (Oct 2017): 4042–49. http://ascopubs.org/doi/abs/10.1200/JCO.2017.74.1363 (accessed Apr 2018).

3. The American Cancer Society Medical and Editorial Content Team, "Survival Rates for Colorectal Cancer, by Stage," *The American Cancer Society* (Feb 2018). https://www.cancer.org/cancer/colon-rectal-cancer/detection -diagnosis-staging/survival-rates.html (accessed Apr 2018).

4. Christopher H. Lieu et al, "Association of Age with Survival in Patients with Metastatic Colorectal Cancer: Analysis from the ARCAD Clinical Trials Program," *Journal of Clinical Oncology* 32.27 (Sep 2014): 2975–82. https:// www.ncbi.nlm.nih.gov/pmc/articles/PMC4809210/ (accessed Apr 2018).

5. Robert Preidt, "Colon Cancer Hits Younger Adults Especially Hard, Study Finds," *HealthDay* (Oct 2013). https://consumer.healthday.com/senior -citizen-information-31/misc-aging-news-10/colon-cancer-hits-younger -adults-especially-hard-study-finds-680634.html (accessed Apr 2018).

6. National Cancer Institute, "Colon Cancer Treatment (PDQ®)–Health Professional Version," *NIH* (Apr 2018). https://www.cancer.gov/types/ colorectal/hp/colon-treatment-pdq#section/all (accessed Apr 2018).

7. Chang Hyun Kim et al, "Prognostic Comparison Between Number and Distribution of Lymph Node Metastases in Patients with Right-Sided Colon

Cancer," *Annals of Surgical Oncology* 21.4 (Apr 2014): 1361–68. https://link .springer.com/article/10.1245/s10434-013-3426-3 (accessed Apr 2018).

8. Robert Preidt, "Colon Cancer's Location May Be Factor in Survival," *WebMD* (2015). https://www.webmd.com/colorectal-cancer/news/20150224/colon -cancers-location-may-be-factor-in-survival (accessed Apr 2018).

9. Fausto Petrelli et al, "Prognostic Survival Associated with Left-Sided vs Right-Sided Colon Cancer: A Systematic Review and Meta-Analysis," *JAMA Oncology* 3.2 (Oct 2017): 211–19. https://www.ncbi.nlm.nih.gov/ pubmed/27787550 (accessed Apr 2018).

CHAPTER 2: Survival of the Sickest

1. Rosalie A. David and Michael R. Zimmerman, "Cancer: An Old Disease, a New Disease or Something in Between?" *Nature Reviews Cancer* 10.10 (Oct 2010): 728–33. https://www.ncbi.nlm.nih.gov/pubmed/20814420 (accessed Apr 2018).

2. William H. Goodson et al, "Assessing the Carcinogenic Potential of Low-Dose Exposures to Chemical Mixtures in the Environment: The Challenge Ahead," *Carcinogenesis* 36.1 (Jun 2015): S254–96. https://www.ncbi.nlm.nih .gov/pmc/articles/PMC4480130/ (accessed Apr 2018).

3. International Agency for Research on Cancer, "IARC: Diesel Engine Exhaust Carcinogenic," *World Health Organization* (Jun 2012). http://www.iarc.fr/en/ media-centre/pr/2012/pdfs/pr213_E.pdf (accessed Apr 2018).

4. Jeffrey Switchenko et al, "Resolving Uncertainty in the Spatial Relationships Between Passive Benzene Exposure and Risk of Non-Hodgkin Lymphoma," *Cancer Epidemiology* 41 (Jul 2016): 139–51. https://www.ncbi.nlm.nih.gov/ pmc/articles/PMC4946246/ (accessed Apr 2018).

5. Goodson et al, "Assessing the Carcinogenic Potential."

6. Michael J. McGinnis and William H. Foege, "The Immediate vs. the Important," *JAMA* 291.10 (Mar 2004): 1263–64. https://jamanetwork.com/ journals/jama/article-abstract/198333 (accessed Apr 2018).

7. Michael J. McGinnis and William H. Foege, "Actual Causes of Death in the United States," *JAMA* 270.18 (Nov 1993): 2207–12. https://jamanetwork .com/journals/jama/article-abstract/409171?redirect=true (accessed Apr 2018).

8. Song Wu et al, "Substantial Contribution of Extrinsic Risk Factors to Cancer Development," *Nature* 529.7584 (Jan 2016): 43–47. https://www.nature.com/ articles/nature16166 (accessed Apr 2018).

9. Doug Irving, "Chronic Conditions in America: Price and Prevalence," *RAND Review* (Jul 2017). https://www.rand.org/blog/rand-review/2017/07/chronic -conditions-in-america-price-and-prevalence.html (accessed Apr 2018).

Endnotes

10. Paul D. Loprinzi et al, "Healthy Lifestyle Characteristics and Their Joint Association with Cardiovascular Disease Biomarkers in US Adults," *Mayo Clinic Proceedings* 91.4 (Apr 2016): 432–42. http://www .mayoclinicproceedings.org/article/S0025-6196%252816%252900043-4/ abstract (accessed Apr 2018).

11. Julie Beck, "Less Than 3 Percent of Americans Live a 'Healthy Lifestyle,'" *The Atlantic* (Mar 2016). https://www.theatlantic.com/health/archive/2016/03/ less-than-3-percent-of-americans-live-a-healthy-lifestyle/475065/ (accessed Apr 2018).

12. Seung Hee Lee-Kwan et al, "Disparities in State-Specific Adult Fruit and Vegetable Consumption—United States, 2015," MMWR 66.45 (Nov 2017): 1241–47. https://www.cdc.gov/mmwr/volumes/66/wr/mm6645a1.htm (accessed Apr 2018).

13. Michael Greger, "Calculate Your Healthy Eating Score," *Nutrition Facts* (Aug 2011). https://nutritionfacts.org/video/calculate-your-healthy-eating-score/ (accessed Apr 2018).

14. M. F. McCarty, "Proposal for a Dietary Phytochemical Index," *Medical Hypotheses* 63.5 (2004): 813–17. https://www.ncbi.nlm.nih.gov/ pubmed/15488652 (accessed 2018).

15. National Cancer Institute, Epidemiology and Genomics Research Program, "Sources of Energy among the U.S. Population, 2005–06," *Epidemiology and Genomics Research Program*. National Cancer Institute (Updated April 2016). http://epi.grants.cancer.gov/diet/foodsources/energy/ (accessed April 2018).

16. Anette Christ et al, "Western Diet Triggers NLRP3-Dependent Innate Immune Reprogramming," *Cell* 172.1–2 (Jan 2018): 162–75.e14. http://www.cell.com/ cell/abstract/S0092-8674(17)31493-9 (accessed Apr 2018).

17. Thibault Fiolet et al, "Consumption of Ultra-Processed Foods and Cancer Risk: Results from NutriNet-Santé Prospective Cohort," *BMJ* 360 (Feb 2018): k322. https://www.bmj.com/content/360/bmj.k322 (accessed Apr 2018).

18. Allison M. Hodge et al, "Consumption of Sugar-Sweetened and Artificially Sweetened Soft Drinks and Risk of Obesity-Related Cancers," *Public Health Nutrition* (Feb 2018): 1–9. https://www.cambridge.org/core/journals/public -health-nutrition/article/consumption-of-sugarsweetened-and-artificially -sweetened-soft-drinks-and-risk-of-obesityrelated-cancers/14DB5E863485356 0209984B07CED68B1 (accessed Apr 2018).

19. Noelle K. LoConte et al, "Alcohol and Cancer: A Statement of the American Society of Clinical Oncology," *Journal of Clinical Oncology* 36.1 (Jan 2018): 83–93. https://www.ncbi.nlm.nih.gov/pubmed/29112463 (accessed Apr 2018).

20. "Millennials 'set to be fattest generation,'" *BBC News* (Feb 2018). http://www .bbc.com/news/health-43195977 (accessed Apr 2018).

21. Centers for Disease Control and Prevention, "Behavioral Risk Factor Surveillance System," *CDC* (reviewed Mar 2018). https://www.cdc.gov/brfss/ (accessed Apr 2018).

22. Brooke C. Steele et al, "Vital Signs: Trends in Incidence of Cancers Associated with Overweight and Obesity—United States, 2005–2014," *Morbidity and Mortality Weekly Report* 66.39 (Oct 2017): 1052–58. https://www.cdc.gov/mmwr/volumes/66/wr/mm6639e1.htm (accessed Apr 2018).

23. Béatrice Lauby-Secretan et al, "Body Fatness and Cancer—Viewpoint of the IARC Working Group," *The New England Journal of Medicine* 375.8 (Aug 2016): 794–98. http://www.nejm.org/doi/full/10.1056/NEJMsr1606602 (accessed Apr 2018).

24. American Association for Cancer Research, "High Body Fat Levels Associated with Increased Breast Cancer Risk in Women with Normal BMI," *ScienceDaily* (Jan 2018) www.sciencedaily.com/releases/2018/01/180126085442.htm (accessed Apr 2018).

25. D. Chakraborty et al, "Fibroblast Growth Factor Receptor Is a Mechanistic Link Between Visceral Adiposity and Cancer," *Oncogene* 36.48 (Nov 2017): 6668–79. https://www.ncbi.nlm.nih.gov/pubmed/28783178 (accessed Apr 2018).

26. C. Stephen et al, "Association of Leisure-Time Physical Activity with Risk of 26 Types of Cancer in 1.44 Million Adults," *JAMA Internal Medicine* 176.6 (Jun 2016): 816–25. https://www.ncbi.nlm.nih.gov/pubmed/27183032 (accessed Apr 2018).

27. Rachel Rettner, "Exercise May Reduce the Risk of These 13 Cancers," *LiveScience* (May 2016). https://www.livescience.com/54749-exercise-reduces-cancer-risk.html (accessed Apr 2018).

28. Center for Nutrition Policy and Promotion, "Nutrient Content of the U.S. Food Supply, 1909–2010," *United States Department of Agriculture* (Mar 2014). https://www.cnpp.usda.gov/USFoodSupply-1909-2010 (accessed Apr 2018).

29. Michael F. Jacobson, "Carcinogenicity and Regulation of Caramel Colorings," *International Journal of Occupational and Environmental Health* 18.3 (Jul–Sep 2012): 254–59. https://www.ncbi.nlm.nih.gov/pubmed/23026009 (accessed Apr 2018).

30. Rudolf Kaaks, "Nutrition, Insulin, IGF-1 Metabolism and Cancer Risk: A Summary of Epidemiological Evidence," *Novartis Foundation Symposium* 262 (2004): 247–60. https://www.ncbi.nlm.nih.gov/pubmed/15562834 (accessed Apr 2018).

31. Samuel S. Epstein, "Re: Role of the Insulin-Like Growth Factors in Cancer Development and Progression," *Journal of the National Cancer Institute* 93.3 (Feb 2001): 238. https://academic.oup.com/jnci/article/93/3/238/2909702 (accessed Apr 2018).

32. American Institute for Cancer Research, "AICR's Foods That Fight Cancer: Whole Grains," *AICR*. http://www.aicr.org/foods-that-fight-cancer/whole -grains.html (accessed Apr 2018).

33. Celine Gasnier et al, "Glyphosate-Based Herbicides Are Toxic and Endocrine Disruptors in Human Cell Line," *Toxicology* 262 (Aug 2009): 184–91. https:// www.ncbi.nlm.nih.gov/pubmed/19539684 (accessed Apr 2018).

34. Anthony Samsel and Stephanie Seneff, "Glyphosate, Pathways to Modern Diseases II: Celiac Sprue and Gluten Intolerance," *Interdisciplinary Toxicology* 6.4 (Dec 2013): 159–84. https://www.ncbi.nlm.nih.gov/pmc/articles/ PMC3945755/ (accessed Apr 2018).

35. Paolo Bofetta, Enzo Merler, and Harri Vainio, "Carcinogenicity of Mercury and Mercury Compounds," *Scandinavian Journal of Work, Environment & Health* 19.1 (Feb 1993): 1–7. https://www.jstor.org/stable/i40043315 (accessed Apr 2018).

36. Environmental Working Group, "First Ever U.S. Tests of Farmed Salmon Show High Levels of Cancer-Causing PCBs," *EWG* (Jul 2003). https://www .ewg.org/news/news-releases/2003/07/30/first-ever-us-tests-farmed-salmon -show-high-levels-cancer-causing-pcbs#.WnDIWiPMw_M (accessed Apr 2018).

37. Mary E. Cogswell et al, "Sodium and Potassium Intakes Among US Adults: NHANES 2003–2008," *American Journal of Clinical Nutrition* 96.3 (Jul 2012): 647–57. https://www.ncbi.nlm.nih.gov/pmc/articles/PMC3417219/ (accessed Apr 2018).

38. Center for Nutrition Policy and Promotion, "Nutrient Content of the U.S. Food Supply, 1909–2010."

39. International Agency for Research on Cancer, "Section of Infections— Infections and Cancer Biology Group," *World Health Organization* (2018). https://www.iarc.fr/en/research-groups/ICB/index.php (accessed Apr 2018).

40. Jeffrey I. Cohen, "Epstein-Barr Virus Vaccines," *Clinical & Translational Immunology* 4.32 (Jan 2015): 1–6. http://www.nature.com/cti/journal/v4/n1/ full/cti201427a.html (accessed Apr 2018).

41. Stephen Starko Francis et al, "In Utero Cytomegalovirus Infection and Development of Childhood Acute Lymphoblastic Leukemia," *Blood* 129.12 (Mar 2017): 1680–84. https://www.ncbi.nlm.nih.gov/pmc/articles/ PMC5364339/ (accessed Apr 2018).

42. "91% of Women Do Not Know about CMV," *National CMV Foundation*. (2018). https://www.nationalcmv.org/home.aspx (accessed Apr 2018).

43. U.S. Department of Agriculture, "Bovine Leukosis Virus (BLV) on U.S. Dairy Operations, 2007," *USDA* (2008). https://www.aphis.usda.gov/animal_ health/nahms/dairy/downloads/dairy07/Dairy07_is_BLV.pdf (accessed Apr 2018).

44. Gertrude Case Buehring et al, "Humans Have Antibodies Reactive with Bovine Leukemia Virus," *AIDS Research and Human Retroviruses* 19.12 (Dec

2003): 1105–13. https://www.ncbi.nlm.nih.gov/pubmed/14709247 (accessed Apr 2018).

45. Gertrude Case Buehring et al, "Exposure to Bovine Leukemia Virus Is Associated with Breast Cancer: A Case-Control Study," *PLoS ONE* 10.9 (Sep 2015): e0134304. http://journals.plos.org/plosone/article?id=10.1371/journal.pone.0134304%20 (accessed Apr 2018).

46. Gertrude Case Buehring et al, "Bovine Leukemia Virus DNA in Human Breast Tissue," *Emerging Infectious Diseases* 20.5 (May 2014): 772–82. https://www.ncbi.nlm.nih.gov/pmc/articles/PMC4012802/ (accessed Apr 2018).

47. Buehring et al, "Exposure to Bovine Leukemia Virus Is Associated with Breast Cancer: A Case-Control Study."

48. D. C. Wilcox et al, "The Okinawan Diet: Health Implications of a Low-Calorie, Nutrient-Dense, Antioxidant-Rich Dietary Pattern Low in Glycemic Load," *The Journal of the American College of Nutrition* 28 (Aug 2009): 500–16. https://www.ncbi.nlm.nih.gov/pubmed/20234038 (accessed Apr 2018).

49. International Agency for Research on Cancer, "GLOBOCAN 2012: Estimated Cancer Incidence, Mortality and Prevalence Worldwide in 2012," *World Health Organization* (2012). http://globocan.iarc.fr (accessed Apr 2018).

50. S. J. O'Keefe et al. "Why Do African Americans Get More Colon Cancer Than Native Africans?" *Journal of Nutrition* 131.1 (Jan 2007): 175–82. https://www.ncbi.nlm.nih.gov/pubmed/17182822 (accessed Apr 2018).

CHAPTER 3: Doctor's Orders

1. Gabrielle Glaser, "Unfortunately, Doctors Are Pretty Good at Suicide," *NCP Journal of Medicine* (Aug 2015). https://www.ncnp.org/journal-of-medicine/1601-unfortunately-doctors-are-pretty-good-at-suicide.html (accessed Apr 2018).

2. Nicholas A. Yaghmour et al, "Causes of Death of Residents in ACGME-Accredited Programs 2000–2014: Implications for the Learning Environment," *Academic Medicine* 92.7 (May 2017): 976–83. https://www.ncbi.nlm.nih.gov/pmc/articles/PMC5483979/ (accessed Apr 2018).

3. Keith H. Berge, Marvin D. Seppala, and Agnes M. Schipper, "Chemical Dependency and the Physician," *Mayo Clinic Proceedings* 84.7 (Jul 2009): 625–31. http://www.mayoclinicproceedings.org/article/S0025-6196(11)60751-9/fulltext (accessed Apr 2018).

4. Barbara Starfield, "Is US Health Really the Best in the World?" *JAMA* 284.4 (Jul 2000): 483–85. https://jamanetwork.com/journals/jama/article-abstract/192908?redirect=true (accessed Apr 2018).

5. Vanessa McMains, "Johns Hopkins Study Suggests Medical Errors Are Third-Leading Cause of Death in U.S.," *HUB* (May 2016). https://hub.jhu.edu/2016/05/03/medical-errors-third-leading-cause-of-death/ (accessed Apr 2018).

Endnotes

6. Donald W. Light, Joel Lexchin, and Jonathan J. Darrow, "Institutional Corruption of Pharmaceuticals and the Myth of Safe and Effective Drugs," *The Journal of Law, Medicine & Ethics* 41.3 (Oct 2013): 590–600. http:// journals.sagepub.com/doi/abs/10.1111/jlme.12068 (accessed Apr 2018).

7. Michael O. Schroeder, "Death by Prescription," *U.S. News & World Report* (Sep 2016). https://health.usnews.com/health-news/patient-advice/ articles/2016-09-27/the-danger-in-taking-prescribed-medications (accessed Apr 2018).

8. John T. James, "A New, Evidence-Based Estimate of Patient Harms Associated with Hospital Care," *Journal of Patient Safety* 9.3 (Sep 2013): 122–28. https:// www.ncbi.nlm.nih.gov/pubmed/23860193 (accessed Apr 2018).

9. Gary Null et al, "Death by Medicine," *WebDC* (2004). http://www.webdc .com/pdfs/deathbymedicine.pdf (accessed Apr 2018).

10. Gary Null et al, "Death by Medicine," *Life Extension Magazine* (2004). http:// www.lifeextension.com/Magazine/2004/3/awsi_death/Page-02 (accessed Apr 2018).

11. Matthew Semler et al, "Balanced Crystalloids versus Saline in Critically Ill Adults," *The New England Journal of Medicine* 378.9 (Mar 2018): 829–839. https://www.nejm.org/doi/full/10.1056/NEJMoa1711584; https://www.ncbi .nlm.nih.gov/pubmed/29485925 (accessed May 2018).

12. Michelle Castillo, "Study Shows Annual Mammograms Don't Save Lives," *CBS News* (Feb 2014). https://www.cbsnews.com/news/canadian-study -shows-annual-mammograms-dont-reduce-breast-cancer-death-rate/ (accessed Apr 2018).

13. Archie Bleyer and H. Gilbert Welch, "Effect of Three Decades of Screening Mammography on Breast-Cancer Incidence," *The New England Journal of Medicine* 367 (Nov 2012): 1998–2005. http://www.nejm.org/doi/full/10.1056/ NEJMoa1206809 (accessed Apr 2018).

14. Louise Davies and H. Gilbert Welch, "Current Thyroid Cancer Trends in the United States," *JAMA Otolaryngology-Head & Neck Surgery* 140.4 (Apr 2014): 317–22. https://jamanetwork.com/journals/jamaotolaryngology/article -abstract/1833060 (accessed Apr 2018).

15. Laura J. Esserman, Ian M. Thompson Jr., and Brian Reid, "Overdiagnosis and Overtreatment in Cancer: An Opportunity for Improvement," *JAMA* 310.8 (Jul 2013): 797–98. https://pdfs.semanticscholar.org/d900/94298f78dd26230 2506473254858060126fb.pdf (accessed Apr 2018).

16. Edward F. Patz et al, "Overdiagnosis in Low-Dose Computed Tomography Screening for Lung Cancer," *JAMA* 174.2 (Jul 2014): 269–74. https://www .ncbi.nlm.nih.gov/pmc/articles/PMC4040004/.

17. Jane C. Weeks et al, "Patients' Expectations about Effects of Chemotherapy for Advanced Cancer," *The New England Journal of Medicine* 367 (Oct 2012):

1616–25. http://www.nejm.org/doi/full/10.1056/NEJMoa1204410 (accessed Apr 2018).

18. Candice M. Wenzell et al, "Outcomes in Obese and Overweight Acute Myeloid Leukemia Patients Receiving Chemotherapy Dosed According to Actual Body Weight," *American Journal of Hematology* 88.10 (Oct 2013): 906–9. https://www.ncbi.nlm.nih.gov/pubmed/23828018 (accessed Apr 2018).

19. Ulrich Abel, "Chemotherapy of Advanced Epithelial Cancer–a Critical Review," *Journal of Biomedicine & Pharmacotherapy* 46.10 (Feb 1992): 439–52. https://www.ncbi.nlm.nih.gov/pubmed/1339108 (accessed Apr 2018).

20. "Lung Cancer Fact Sheet," *American Lung Association* (2016), http://www.lung.org/lung-health-and-diseases/lung-disease-lookup/lung-cancer/resource-library/lung-cancer-fact-sheet.html (accessed Apr 2018).

21. National Cancer Institute, "SEER Cancer Statistics Review, 1975–2013," *NIH* (Sep 2016). https://seer.cancer.gov/archive/csr/1975_2013/ (accessed Apr 2018).

22. Hesborn Wao et al, "Survival of Patients with Non–Small Cell Lung Cancer Without Treatment: A Systematic Review and Meta-Analysis," *Systematic Reviews* 2 (Feb 2013): 10. https://www.ncbi.nlm.nih.gov/pmc/articles/PMC3579762/ (accessed Apr 2018).

23. N. Bernards et al, "No Improvement in Median Survival for Patients with Metastatic Gastric Cancer Despite Increased Use of Chemotherapy," *Annals of Oncology* 24.12 (Dec 2013): 3056–60. https://academic.oup.com/annonc/article/24/12/3056/172397 (accessed Apr 2018).

24. Holly G. Prigerson et al, "Chemotherapy Use, Performance Status, and Quality of Life at the End of Life," *JAMA Oncology* 1.6 (Jul 2015): 778–84. https://www.ncbi.nlm.nih.gov/pubmed/26203912 (accessed Apr 2018).

CHAPTER 4: Making a Killing

1. R. Jeffrey Smith and Jeffrey H. Birnbaum, "Drug Bill Demonstrates Lobby's Pull," *Washington Post* (Jan 2007). http://www.washingtonpost.com/wp-dyn/content/article/2007/01/11/AR2007011102081.html (accessed Apr 2018).

2. Gardiner Harris, "Waste in Cancer Drugs Costs $3 Billion a Year, a Study Says," *The New York Times* (Mar 2016). https://www.nytimes.com/2016/03/01/health/waste-in-cancer-drugs-costs-3-billion-a-year-a-study-says.html (accessed Apr 2018).

3. Jackie Judd, "Taxpayers End Up Funding Drug Companies," *ABC News* (Jun 2012). http://abcnews.go.com/WNT/YourMoney/story?id=129651 (accessed Apr 2018).

4. M. D. Kesselheim et al, "The High Cost of Prescription Drugs in the United States Origins and Prospects for Reform," *JAMA* 316.8 (Aug 2016): 858–71. https://www.ncbi.nlm.nih.gov/pubmed/27552619 (accessed Apr 2018).

5. Marcia Angell, "Drug Companies and Doctors: A Story of Corruption," *The New York Review of Books* (Jan 2009). http://www.nybooks.com/articles/archives/2009/jan/15/drug-companies-doctorsa-story-of-corruption/ (accessed Apr 2018).

6. Centers for Disease Control and Prevention, "Prescription Painkiller Overdoses in the US," *CDC* (Nov 2011). http://www.cdc.gov/vitalsigns/PainkillerOverdoses/index.html (accessed Apr 2018).

7. Irving Kirsch, "Antidepressants and the Placebo Effect," *Zeitschrift Für Psychologie* 222.3 (2014): 128–34. https://www.ncbi.nlm.nih.gov/pmc/articles/PMC4172306/ (accessed Apr 2018).

8. C. Glenn Begley and Lee M. Ellis, "Drug Development: Raise Standards for Preclinical Cancer Research," *Nature* 483 (Mar 2012): 531–33. https://www.ncbi.nlm.nih.gov/pubmed/22460880 (accessed Apr 2018).

9. Sharon Begley, "In Cancer Science, Many 'Discoveries' Don't Hold Up," *Reuters* (Mar 2012). https://www.reuters.com/article/us-science-cancer/in-cancer-science-many-discoveries-dont-hold-up-idUSBRE82R12P20120328 (accessed Apr 2018).

10. Florian Prinz, Thomas Schlange, and Khusru Asadullah, "Believe It or Not: How Much Can We Rely on Published Data on Potential Drug Targets?" *Nature Reviews Drug Discovery* 10.9 (Aug 2011): 712. http://www.nature.com/articles/nrd3439-c1 (accessed Apr 2018).

11. Daniele Mandrioli, Cristin E Kearns, and Lisa A. Bero, "Relationship Between Research Outcomes and Risk of Bias, Study Sponsorship, and Author Financial Conflicts of Interest in Reviews of the Effects of Artificially Sweetened Beverages on Weight Outcomes: A Systematic Review of Reviews," *PLoS ONE* 11.9 (Sep 2016): e0162198. http://journals.plos.org/plosone/article?id=10.1371/journal.pone.0162198 (accessed Apr 2018).

12. C. Ferric et al, "Misconduct Accounts for the Majority of Retracted Scientific Publications," *Proceedings of the National Academy of Sciences* 109.42 (Sep 2012): 17028–33. http://www.pnas.org/content/109/42/17028 (accessed Apr 2018).

13. Richard Horton, "Offline: What Is Medicine's 5 Sigma?" *The Lancet* 385.9976 (Apr 2015): 1380. http://www.thelancet.com/journals/lancet/article/PIIS0140-6736(15)60696-1/fulltext (accessed Apr 2018).

14. Angell, "Drug Companies and Doctors: A Story of Corruption."

15. Hope S. Rugo et al, "Randomized Phase III Trial of Paclitaxel Once Per Week Compared With Nanoparticle Albumin-Bound Nab-Paclitaxel Once Per Week or Ixabepilone With Bevacizumab As First-Line Chemotherapy for Locally Recurrent or Metastatic Breast Cancer: CALGB 40502/NCCTG N063H (Alliance)," *Journal of Clinical Oncology* 33.21 (2014): 2361–69. https://www.ncbi.nlm.nih.gov/pubmed/26056183 (accessed Apr 2018).

16. "Study Confirms Taxol Better Than Ixempra or Abraxane for Locally Advanced or Metastatic Disease," *BreastCancer.org* (Jun 2015). http://www .breastcancer.org/research-news/taxol-better-than-ixempra-or-abraxane (accessed Apr 2018).

17. Courtney Davis et al, "Availability of Evidence of Benefits on Overall Survival and Quality of Life of Cancer Drugs Approved by European Medicines Agency: Retrospective Cohort Study of Drug Approvals 2009–13," *BMJ* 359 (Oct 2017). https://www.bmj.com/content/359/bmj.j4530 (accessed Apr 2018).

18. "No Clear Evidence That Most New Cancer Drugs Extend or Improve Life." *BMJ Newsroom* (Oct 2017). http://www.bmj.com/company/newsroom/ no-clear-evidence-that-most-new-cancer-drugs-extend-or-improve-life/ (accessed Apr 2018).

19. Margaret Hamburg, "FDA Pulls Approval for Avastin in Breast Cancer," *Cancer Discovery* (Nov 2011). http://cancerdiscovery.aacrjournals.org/ content/candisc/early/2011/11/21/2159-8290.CD-ND112311OL-08.full.pdf (accessed Apr 2018).

20. Vishal Ranpura, Sanjaykumar Hapani, and Shenhong Wu, "Treatment-Related Mortality with Bevacizumab in Cancer Patients: A Meta-Analysis," *JAMA* 305.5 (2011): 487–94. https://jamanetwork.com/journals/jama/ fullarticle/645368 (accessed Apr 2018).

21. National Cancer Institute, "When Combined with Chemotherapy, Bevacizumab Is Associated with Increased Risk of Death," *NCI* (Mar 2011). https://www.cancer.gov/types/colorectal/research/bevacizumab-severe-side -effects (accessed Apr 2018).

22. Ed Silverman, "Drug Makers Pay $67 Million for Misleading Docs About Cancer Drug Survival Data," *STAT News* (Jun 2016). https://www.statnews .com/pharmalot/2016/06/06/drug-makers-pay-67m-misleading-docs-cancer -drug-survival-data/ (accessed Apr 2018).

23. Office of Public Affairs, "Pharmaceutical Companies to Pay $67 Million To Resolve False Claims Act Allegations Relating to Tarceva," *United States Department of Justice* (Jun 2016). https://www.justice.gov/opa/pr/ pharmaceutical-companies-pay-67-million-resolve-false-claims-act -allegations-relating-tarceva (accessed Apr 2018).

24. Graeme Morgan, Robyn Ward and Michael Barton, "The Contribution of Cytotoxic Chemotherapy to 5-Year Survival in Adult Malignancies," *Journal of Clinical Oncology* 16.8 (2004): 549–60. http://www.clinicaloncologyonline .net/article/S0936-6555(04)00222-5/abstract (accessed Apr 2018).

25. Chris Kahlenborn et al, "Oral Contraceptive Use as a Risk Factor for Premenopausal Breast Cancer: A Meta-Analysis," *Mayo Clinic Proceedings* 81.10 (Oct 2006): 1290–302. https://www.ncbi.nlm.nih.gov/ pubmed/17036554 (accessed Apr 2018).

Endnotes

26. Yu Sun et al, "Treatment-Induced Damage to the Tumor Microenvironment Promotes Prostate Cancer Therapy Resistance Through WNT16B," *Nature Medicine* 18.9 (Sep 2012): 1359–68. https://www.ncbi.nlm.nih.gov/pmc/articles/PMC3677971/ (accessed Apr 2018).

27. Beth Israel Deaconess Medical Center, "Double-Edged Sword: Killing Cancer Cells Can Also Drive Tumor Growth," *EurekAlert!* (Nov 2017). https://www.eurekalert.org/pub_releases/2017-11/bidm-dsk113017.php (accessed Apr 2018).

28. Gali Weinreb, "Research: Chemotherapy Can Cause Metastasis," *Globes* (Dec 2016). http://www.globes.co.il/en/article-technion-research-finds-chemotherapy-can-cause-metastasis-1001164952 (accessed Apr 2018).

29. Fred Hutchinson Cancer Research Center, "Long-Term Tamoxifen Use Increases Risk of an Aggressive, Hard to Treat Type of Second Breast Cancer," *ScienceDaily* (Aug 2009). https://www.sciencedaily.com/releases/2009/08/090825150954.htm (accessed Apr 2018).

30. Christina Izzo, "Weighing the Risks and Benefits of Tamoxifen as Chemoprevention in High-Risk Women," *Cancer Updates, Research & Education* (Jan 2015). https://www.curetoday.com/articles/weighing-the-risks-and-benefits-of-tamoxifen-as-chemoprevention-in-high-risk-women (accessed Apr 2018).

31. Shezad Malik, "Taxotere Permanent Hair Loss Lawsuit," *The Legal Examiner* (Mar 2016). http://fortworth.legalexaminer.com/fda-prescription-drugs/taxotere-permanent-hair-loss-lawsuit/ (accessed Apr 2018).

32. Nathan Gay and Vinay Prasad, "Few People Actually Benefit from 'Breakthrough' Cancer Immunotherapy," *STAT News* (Mar 2017). https://www.statnews.com/2017/03/08/immunotherapy-cancer-breakthrough/ (accessed Apr 2018).

33. James Larkin, "Combined Nivolumab and Ipilimumab or Monotherapy in Untreated Melanoma," *The New England Journal of Medicine* 373.1 (Jul 2015): 23–34. http://www.nejm.org/doi/full/10.1056/NEJMoa1504030 (accessed Apr 2018).

34. Zosia Chustecka, "New Immunotherapy Costing $1 Million a Year," *Medscape* (Jun 2015). https://www.medscape.com/viewarticle/845707 (accessed Apr 2018).

35. Megan Molteni, "The Most Promising Cancer Treatments in a Century Have Arrived—but Not for Everyone," *Wired* (Nov 2017). https://www.wired.com/story/cancer-immunotherapy-has-arrived-but-not-for-everyone/ (accessed Apr 2018).

36. Janet M. Busey et al, "Patient Knowledge and Understanding of Radiation from Diagnostic Imaging," *JAMA Internal Medicine* 173.3 (Feb 2013): 239–41. https://jamanetwork.com/journals/jamainternalmedicine/fullarticle/1487286 (accessed Apr 2018).

37. "Radiation Dose in X-Ray and CT Exams," *Radiology Info* (Feb 2017). https://www.radiologyinfo.org/en/info.cfm?pg=safety-xray (accessed Apr 2018).

38. Andrew J. Einstein, "Beyond the Bombs: Cancer Risks from Low-Dose Medical Radiation," *Lancet* 380.9840 (Jun 2012): 455–57. https://www.ncbi.nlm.nih.gov/pmc/articles/PMC3674023/ (accessed Apr 2018).

39. Amy Berrington de Gonzalez et al, "Projected Cancer Risks from Computed Tomographic Scans Performed in the United States in 2007," *JAMA Internal Medicine* 169.22 (Dec 2009): 2071–77. https://www.ncbi.nlm.nih.gov/pubmed/20008689 (accessed Apr 2018).

40. David B. Larson et al, "Rising Use of CT in Child Visits to the Emergency Department in the United States, 1995–2008," *Radiology* 259.3 (Jun 2011): 793–801. https://www.ncbi.nlm.nih.gov/pubmed/21467249 (accessed Apr 2018).

41. Mark S. Pearce, "Radiation Exposure from CT Scans in Childhood and Subsequent Risk of Leukaemia and Brain Tumours: A Retrospective Cohort Study," *Lancet* 380.9840 (Aug 2012): 499–505. http://www.thelancet.com/journals/lancet/article/PIIS0140-6736(12)60815-0/abstract (accessed Apr 2018).

42. Geoffrey R. Oxnard et al, "Variability of Lung Tumor Measurements on Repeat Computed Tomography Scans Taken Within 15 Minutes," *Journal of Clinical Oncology* 29.23 (Jul 2011): 3114–19. https://www.ncbi.nlm.nih.gov/pmc/articles/PMC3157977/ (accessed Apr 2018).

43. Carrie Printz, "Radiation Treatment Generates Therapy-Resistant Cancer Stem Cells from Less Aggressive Breast Cancer Cells," *Cancer* 118.13 (Jun 2012): 3225. https://onlinelibrary.wiley.com/doi/full/10.1002/cncr.27701 (accessed Apr 2018).

44. Chann Lagadec et al, "Radiation-Induced Reprogramming of Breast Cancer Cells," *Stem Cells* 30.5 (May 2012): 833–44. https://www.ncbi.nlm.nih.gov/pmc/articles/PMC3413333/ (accessed Apr 2018).

45. Syed Wamique Yusuf, Shehzad Sami, and Iyad N. Daher, "Radiation-Induced Heart Disease: A Clinical Update," *Cardiology Research and Practice* 2011 (Dec 2010): 317659. https://www.hindawi.com/journals/crp/2011/317659/ (accessed Apr 2018).

46. Manisha Palta et al, "The Use of Adjuvant Radiotherapy in Elderly Patients with Early-Stage Breast Cancer: Changes in Practice Patterns After Publication of Cancer and Leukemia Group B 9343," *Cancer* 121.2 (Jan 2015): 188–93. https://www.ncbi.nlm.nih.gov/pubmed/25488523 (accessed Apr 2018).

47. Elizabeth B. Claus et al, "Dental X-Rays and Risk of Meningioma," *Cancer* 118.18 (Apr 2012): 4530–37. https://www.ncbi.nlm.nih.gov/pmc/articles/PMC3396782/ (accessed Apr 2018).

48. American Dental Association Council on Scientific Affairs, "The Use of Dental Radiographs: Update and Recommendations." *Journal of the American Dental Association* 137.9 (Sep 2006): 1304–12. http://jada.ada.org/article/ S0002-8177(14)64322-1/fulltext (accessed Apr 2018).

CHAPTER 5: It's Not Like I Need Your Business

1. Louis S. Goodman et al, "Nitrogen Mustard Therapy: Use of Methyl-Bis(Beta-Chloroethyl)amine Hydrochloride and Tris(Beta-Chloroethyl) amine Hydrochloride for Hodgkin's Disease, Lymphosarcoma, Leukemia and Certain Allied and Miscellaneous Disorders," *JAMA* 132.3 (Sep 1946): 126–32. https://jamanetwork.com/journals/jama/article -abstract/288442?redirect=true (accessed Apr 2018).

2. Tom Reynolds, "Salary a Major Factor for Academic Oncologists, Study Shows," *Journal of the National Cancer Institute* 93.7 (Apr 2001): 491. https:// academic.oup.com/jnci/article/93/7/491/2906507 (accessed Apr 2108).

3. Mireille Jacobsone et al, "How Medicare's Payment Cuts for Cancer Chemotherapy Drugs Changed Patterns of Treatment," *Health Affairs* 29.7 (Jul 2010): 1394–402. https://www.healthaffairs.org/doi/abs/10.1377/ hlthaff.2009.0563 (accessed Apr 2018).

4. Jean M. Mitchell, "Urologists' Use of Intensity-Modulated Radiation Therapy for Prostate Cancer," *New England Journal of Medicine* 369.17 (Oct 2013): 1629–637. http://www.nejm.org/doi/full/10.1056/NEJMsa1201141 (accessed Apr 2018).

5. Lee N. Newcomer, "Changing Physician Incentives for Affordable, Quality Cancer Care: Results of an Episode Payment Model." *Journal of Oncology Practice* 10 (Jul 2014): 322–26. http://ascopubs.org/doi/abs/10.1200/ jop.2014.001488 (accessed Apr 2018).

6. Matthew Herper, "The Truly Staggering Cost of Inventing New Drugs," *Forbes* (Feb 2012). https://www.forbes.com/sites/matthewherper/2012/02/10/the -truly-staggering-cost-of-inventing-new-drugs/#41ee3fa44a94 (accessed Apr 2018).

7. Rosie Taylor and Jim Giles, "Cash Interests Taint Drug Advice," *Nature* 437 (Oct 2005): 1070–71. http://www.nature.com/articles/4371070a (accessed Apr 2018).

8. Caroline Riveros et al, "Timing and Completeness of Trial Results Posted at ClinicalTrials.gov and Published in Journals," *PLoS Medicine* 10.12 (Dec 2013): e1001566. http://journals.plos.org/plosmedicine/article?id=10.1371/ journal.pmed.1001566 (accessed Apr 2018).

9. Bob Grant, "Merck Published Fake Journal," *The Scientist Magazine* (Apr 2009). https://www.the-scientist.com/?articles.view/articleNo/27376/title/ Merck-published-fake-journal/ (accessed Apr 2018).

10. Jim Edwards, "Merck Created Hit List to 'Destroy,' 'Neutralize' or 'Discredit' Dissenting Doctors," *CBS News* (May 2009). https://www.cbsnews.com/news/merck-created-hit-list-to-destroy-neutralize-or-discredit-dissenting-doctors/ (accessed Apr 2018).

11. Laura B. Vater et al, "Trends in Cancer-Center Spending on Advertising in the United States, 2005 to 2014," *JAMA Internal Medicine* 176.8 (Aug 2016): 1214–16. https://jamanetwork.com/journals/jamainternalmedicine/fullarticle/2532786 (accessed Apr 2018).

12. Laura B. Vater et al, "What Are Cancer Centers Advertising to the Public?: A Content Analysis," *Annals of Internal Medicine* 160.12 (Jun 2014): 813–20. https://www.ncbi.nlm.nih.gov/pmc/articles/PMC4356527/ (accessed Apr 2018).

13. Scott D. Ramsey et al, "Washington State Cancer Patients Found to Be at Greater Risk for Bankruptcy Than People without a Cancer Diagnosis," *Health Affairs* 32.6 (May 2013): 1143–52. https://www.ncbi.nlm.nih.gov/pmc/articles/PMC4240626/ (accessed Apr 2018).

CHAPTER 6: The Elephant in the Waiting Room

1. Michael J. Thun and Ahmedin Jemal, "How Much of the Decrease in Cancer Death Rates in the United States Is Attributable to Reductions in Tobacco Smoking?" *Tobacco Control* 15.5 (Oct 2006): 345–47. https://www.ncbi.nlm.nih.gov/pmc/articles/PMC2563648/ (accessed Apr 2018).

2. Peter M. Ravdin et al, "The Decrease in Breast-Cancer Incidence in 2003 in the United States," *The New England Journal of Medicine* 356.16 (Apr 2007): 1670–74. http://www.nejm.org/doi/full/10.1056/NEJMsr070105 (accessed Apr 2018).

3. Collaborative Group on Epidemiological Studies of Ovarian Cancer, "Menopausal Hormone Use and Ovarian Cancer Risk: Individual Participant Meta-Analysis of 52 Epidemiological Studies," *The Lancet* 385.9980 (May 2015): 1835–42. https://www.ncbi.nlm.nih.gov/pubmed/25684585 (accessed Apr 2018).

4. Odette Wegwarth, Wolfgang Gaissmaier, and Gerd Gigerenzer, "Deceiving Numbers: Survival Rates and Their Impact on Doctors' Risk Communication," *Medical Decision Making* 31.3 (Dec 2010): 386–94. http://journals.sagepub.com/doi/abs/10.1177/0272989X10391469 (accessed Apr 2018).

5. Steven A. Narod et al, "Breast Cancer Mortality After a Diagnosis of Ductal Carcinoma in Situ," *JAMA Oncology* 1.7 (Oct 2015): 888–96. https://www.ncbi.nlm.nih.gov/pubmed/26291673 (accessed Apr 2018).

6. Allison W. Kurian, "Recent Trends in Chemotherapy Use and Oncologists' Treatment Recommendations for Early-Stage Breast Cancer," *Journal of the National Cancer Institute* (Dec 2017): djx239. http://ascopubs.org/doi/abs/10.1200/JCO.2017.35.15_suppl.541 (accessed Apr 2018).

7. Fatima Cardoso et al. "70-Gene Signature as an Aid to Treatment Decisions in Early-Stage Breast Cancer," *The New England Journal of Medicine* 375 (Aug 2016): 717–29. http://www.nejm.org/doi/full/10.1056/NEJMoa1602253 (accessed Apr 2018).

CHAPTER 8: Plants versus Zombies

1. William W. Li et al, "Tumor Angiogenesis as a Target for Dietary Cancer Prevention," *Journal of Oncology* 2012 (Jul 2011): 1–23. https://www.hindawi.com/journals/jo/2012/879623/ (accessed Apr 2018).

2. Jie Sun et al, "Antioxidant and Antiproliferative Activities of Common Fruits," *Journal of Agricultural and Food Chemistry* 50.25 (Dec 2002): 7449–54. https://www.ncbi.nlm.nih.gov/pubmed/12452674 (accessed Apr 2018).

3. Katherine M. Weh, Jennifer Clarke, and Laura A. Kresty, "Cranberries and Cancer: An Update of Preclinical Studies Evaluating the Cancer Inhibitory Potential of Cranberry and Cranberry Derived Constituents," *Antioxidants* 5.3 (Aug 2016): 27. https://www.ncbi.nlm.nih.gov/pmc/articles/PMC5039576/ (accessed Apr 2018).

4. Navindra P. Seeram et al, "Total Cranberry Extract versus Its Phytochemical Constituents: Antiproliferative and Synergistic Effects against Human Tumor Cell Lines," *Journal of Agricultural and Food Chemistry* 52.9 (Apr 2004): 2512–17. https://pubs.acs.org/doi/abs/10.1021/jf0352778 (accessed Apr 2018).

5. Lisa S. McAnulty et al, "Effect of Blueberry Ingestion on Natural Killer Cell Counts, Oxidative Stress, and Inflammation Prior To and After 2.5 H of Running," *Applied Physiology, Nutrition, and Metabolism* 36.6 (Nov 2011): 976–84. http://www.nrcresearchpress.com/doi/abs/10.1139/h11-120#.Ws0H47CG-hc (accessed Apr 2018).

6. Gordon J. McDougall, "Extracts Exert Different Antiproliferative Effects against Cervical and Colon Cancer Cells Grown In Vitro," *Journal of Agricultural and Food Chemistry* 56.9 (Apr 2008): 3016–23. https://www.ncbi.nlm.nih.gov/pubmed/18412361 (accessed Apr 2018).

7. Marie E. Olsson et al, "Antioxidant Levels and Inhibition of Cancer Cell Proliferation In Vitro by Extracts from Organically and Conventionally Cultivated Strawberries," *Journal of Agricultural and Food Chemistry* 54.4 (Feb 2006): 1248–55. https://www.ncbi.nlm.nih.gov/pubmed/16478244 (accessed Apr 2018).

8. Chen, Tong et al, "Randomized Phase II Trial of Lyophilized Strawberries in Patients with Dysplastic Precancerous Lesions of the Esophagus," *Cancer Prevention Research* 5.1 (Jan 2012): 41–50. https://www.ncbi.nlm.nih.gov/pubmed/22135048 (accessed Apr 2018).

9. Brian S. Shumway et al, "Effects of a Topically Applied Bioadhesive Berry Gel on Loss of Heterozygosity Indices in Premalignant Oral Lesions," *Cancer Prevention Research* 14.8 (Nov 2008): 2421–30. https://www.ncbi.nlm.nih.gov/pmc/articles/PMC3498466/ (accessed Apr 2018).

10. C. Ngamkitidechakul et al, "Antitumour Effects of Phyllanthus emblica L.: Induction of Cancer Cell Apoptosis and Inhibition of In Vivo Tumour Promotion and In Vitro Invasion of Human Cancer Cells," *Phytotherapy Research* 24.9 (Sep 2010): 1405–13. https://www.ncbi.nlm.nih.gov/pubmed/20812284 (accessed Apr 2018).

11. Muhammad S. Akhtar, "Effect of Amla Fruit (Emblica officinalis Gaertn.) on Blood Glucose and Lipid Profile of Normal Subjects and Type 2 Diabetic Patients," *International Journal of Food Sciences and Nutrition* 62.6 (Apr 2011): 609-616. https://www.ncbi.nlm.nih.gov/pubmed/21495900 (accessed Apr 2018).

12. Dominique Boivin et al, "Antiproliferative and Antioxidant Activities of Common Vegetables: A Comparative Study," *Food Chemistry* 112.2 (Jan 2009): 374–80. https://www.sciencedirect.com/science/article/pii/S0308814608006419 (accessed Apr 2018).

13. Yi-Fang Chu et al, "Antioxidant and Antiproliferative Activities of Common Vegetables," *Journal of Agricultural and Food Chemistry* 50.23 (Dec 2002): 6910–16. https://www.researchgate.net/publication/8665499_Antioxidant_and_Antiproliferative_Activities_of_Common_Vegetables (accessed Apr 2018).

14. Cai-Xia Zhang et al, "Greater Vegetable and Fruit Intake Is Associated with a Lower Risk of Breast Cancer Among Chinese Women," *International Journal of Cancer* 125.1 (Jul 2009): 181 –88. (Zhang) https://www.ncbi.nlm.nih.gov/pubmed/19358284 (accessed Apr 2018).

15. Victoria A. Kirsh et al, "Prospective Study of Fruit and Vegetable Intake and Risk of Prostate Cancer," *Journal of the National Cancer Institute* 99.15 (Aug 2007): 1200–1209. https://www.ncbi.nlm.nih.gov/pubmed/17652276 (accessed Apr 2018).

16. Shiuan Chen et al, "Anti-Aromatase Activity of Phytochemicals in White Button Mushrooms (Agaricus bisporus)," *Cancer Research* 66.24 (Dec 2006): 12026–34. https://www.ncbi.nlm.nih.gov/pubmed/17178902 (accessed Apr 2018).

17. Sang Chul Jeong, Sundar Rao Koyyalamudi, and Gerald Pang, "Dietary Intake of *Agaricus bisporus* White Button Mushroom Accelerates Salivary Immunoglobulin A Secretion in Healthy Volunteers," *Nutrition* 28.5 (May 2012): 527–31. http://www.nutritionjrnl.com/article/S0899-9007(11)00302-9/abstract (accessed Apr 2018).

18. N. N. Miura et al, "Blood Clearance of (1-->3)-beta-D-glucan in MRL lpr/lpr Mice," *FEMS Immunology and Medical Microbiology* 13.1 (Feb 1996): 51–57. https://www.researchgate.net/publication/14384731_Blood_clearance_of_1--3-beta-D-glucan_in_MRL_lprlpr_mice (accessed Apr 2018).

19. David C. Nieman, "Exercise Effects on Systemic Immunity," *Immunology and Cell Biology* 78.5 (Oct 2000): 496–501. https://www.researchgate.net/publication/274166266_Exercise_effects_on_systemic_immunity (accessed Apr 2018).

Endnotes

20. Min Zhang et al, "Dietary Intakes of Mushrooms and Green Tea Combine to Reduce the Risk of Breast Cancer in Chinese Women," *International Journal of Cancer* 124.6 (Mar 2008): 1404–8. https://www.ncbi.nlm.nih.gov/pubmed/19048616 (accessed Apr 2018).

21. Amanda Hutchins-Wolfbrandt and Anahita M. Mistry, "Dietary Turmeric Potentially Reduces the Risk of Cancer," *Asian Pacific Journal of Cancer Prevention* 12.12 (Jan 2011): 3169–73. https://www.researchgate.net/publication/223984006_Dietary_Turmeric_Potentially_Reduces_the_Risk_of_Cancer (accessed Apr 2018).

22. S. Bengmark, M. D. Mesa, and A. Gil, "Plant-Derived Health: The Effects of Turmeric and Curcuminoids," *Nutrición Hospitalaria* 24.3 (May–Jun 2009): 273–81. https://www.ncbi.nlm.nih.gov/pubmed/19721899 (accessed Apr 2018).

23. Noor Hasima and Bharat B. Aggarwal, "Cancer-Linked Targets Modulated by Curcumin," *International Journal of Biochemistry and Molecular Biology* 3.4 (Dec 2012): 328–51. https://www.ncbi.nlm.nih.gov/pmc/articles/PMC3533886/ (accessed Apr 2018).

24. Bharat B. Aggarwal, A. Kumar, and A. C. Bharti, "Anticancer Potential of Curcumin: Preclinical and Clinical Studies," *Anticancer Research* 23.1a (Jan–Feb 2003): 363–98. https://www.ncbi.nlm.nih.gov/pubmed/12680238 (accessed Apr 2018).

25. Christopher D. Lao et al, "Dose Escalation of a Curcuminoid Formulation," *BMC Complementary and Alternative Medicine* 6:10 (Feb 2006). https://www.researchgate.net/publication/7234027_Dose_escalation_of_a_curcuminoid_formulation_BMC_Complement_Altern_Med_610 (accessed Apr 2018).

26. Subash C. Gupta, Sridevi Patchva, and Bharat B. Aggarwal, "Therapeutic Roles of Curcumin: Lessons Learned from Clinical Trials," *The AAPS Journal* 15.1 (Jan 2013): 195–218. https://www.ncbi.nlm.nih.gov/pmc/articles/PMC3535097/ (accessed Apr 2018).

27. Abbas Zaidi, Maggie Lai, and Jamie Cavenagh, "Long-Term Stabilisation of Myeloma with Curcumin," *BMJ Case Reports* 2017 (Apr 2017). http://casereports.bmj.com/content/2017/bcr-2016-218148.abstract (accessed Apr 2018).

28. Guido Shoba et al, "Influence of Piperine on the Pharmacokinetics of Curcumin in Animals and Human Volunteers," *Planta Medica* 64.4 (May 1998): 353–56. https://www.ncbi.nlm.nih.gov/pubmed/96191201 (accessed Apr 2018).

29. I. Savini et al, "Origanum vulgare Induces Apoptosis in Human Colon Cancer Caco2 Cells," *Nutrition and Cancer* 61.3 (Feb 2009): 381–89. https://www.researchgate.net/publication/24284438_Origanum_Vulgare_Induces_Apoptosis_in_Human_Colon_Cancer_Caco_2_Cells (accessed Apr 2018).

30. Ladislav Vaško et al, "Comparison of Some Antioxidant Properties of Plant Extracts from Origanum vulgare, Salvia officinalis, Eleutherococcus senticosus

and Stevia rebaudiana," *In Vitro Cellular & Developmental Biology—Animal* 50.7 (Aug 2014): 614–22. https://www.ncbi.nlm.nih.gov/pubmed/24737278 (accessed Apr 2018).

31. Federation of American Societies for Experimental Biology (FASEB), "Component of Pizza Seasoning Herb Oregano Kills Prostate Cancer Cells," *ScienceDaily* (Apr 2012). www.sciencedaily.com/ releases/2012/04/120424162224.htm (accessed Apr 2018).

32. National Cancer Institute, "Garlic and Cancer Prevention," (Jan 2008). https://www.cancer.gov/about-cancer/causes-prevention/risk/diet/garlic-fact -sheet (accessed Apr 2018).

33. Shunsuke Kimura, "Black Garlic: A Critical Review of Its Production, Bioactivity, and Application," *Journal of Food and Drug Analysis* 25.1 (Jan 2017): 62–70. https://www.sciencedirect.com/science/article/pii/ S1021949816301727 (accessed Apr 2018).

34. Ruth Clark and Seong-Ho Lee, "Anticancer Properties of Capsaicin Against Human Cancer," *Anticancer Research* 36.3 (Feb 2016): 837–43. http:// ar.iiarjournals.org/content/36/3/837.abstract (accessed Apr 2018).

35. Kristin L. Kamerud, Kevin A. Hobbie, and Kim A. Anderson. "Stainless Steel Leaches Nickel and Chromium into Foods During Cooking," *Journal of Agriculture and Food Chemistry* 61.39 (Aug 2013): 9495–501. https://pubs.acs .org/doi/abs/10.1021/jf402400v (accessed Apr 2018).

36. Dugald Seely et al, "In Vitro Analysis of the Herbal Compound Essiac," *Anticancer Research* 27.6b (Nov–Dec 2007): 3875–82. https://www.ncbi.nlm .nih.gov/pubmed/18225545 (accessed Apr 2018).

37. Yan Sun et al, "Immune Restoration and/or Augmentation of Local Graft versus Host Reaction by Traditional Chinese Medicinal Herbs," *Cancer* 52.1 (Jul 1983): 70–73. https://www.ncbi.nlm.nih.gov/pubmed/6336578 (accessed Apr 2018).

38. Yan San et al, "Herbaline—(Special Spice)," *Jason Winters International.* https://sirjasonwinters.com/scientific-documentation-herbalene/ (accessed Apr 2018).

39. Jian-Ming Lü et al, "Molecular Mechanisms and Clinical Applications of Nordihydroguaiaretic Acid (NDGA) and Its Derivatives: An Update," *Medical Science Monitor* 16.5 (Aug 2010): RA93–100. https://www.ncbi.nlm.nih.gov/ pmc/articles/PMC2927326/ (accessed Apr 2018).

40. Xiaoxia Li et al, "A Review of Recent Research Progress on the Astragalus Genus," *Molecules* 19.11 (Nov 2014): 18850–80. https://www.ncbi.nlm.nih .gov/pubmed/25407722 (accessed Apr 2018).

41. Arash Khorasani Esmaeili et al, "Antioxidant Activity and Total Phenolic and Flavonoid Content of Various Solvent Extracts from In Vivo and In Vitro Grown Trifolium pratense L. (Red Clover)," *BioMed Research*

International 2015 (Apr 2015): 643285. https://www.hindawi.com/journals/bmri/2015/643285/ (accessed Apr 2018).

42. Yun Wang et al, "The Red Clover (Trifolium pratense) Isoflavone Biochanin A Inhibits Aromatase Activity and Expression," *British Journal of Nutrition* 99.2 (May 2008): 303–10. https://www.researchgate.net/publication/6079305_The_red_clover_Trifolium_pratense_isoflavone_biochanin_A_inhibits_aromatase_activity_and_expression (accessed Apr 2018).

43. Pamela Ovadje et al, "Dandelion Root Extract Affects Colorectal Cancer Proliferation and Survival Through the Activation of Multiple Death Signalling Pathways," *Oncotarget* 7.45 (Nov 2016): 73080–100. https://www.ncbi.nlm.nih.gov/pmc/articles/PMC5341965/ (accessed Apr 2018).

44. Sophia C. Sigstedt et al, "Evaluation of Aqueous Extracts of Taraxacum officinale on Growth and Invasion of Breast and Prostate Cancer Cells," *International Journal of Oncology* 32.5 (May 2008): 1085–90. https://www.ncbi.nlm.nih.gov/pubmed/18425335 (accessed Apr 2018).

45. Pamela Ovadje et al, "Selective Induction of Apoptosis Through Activation of Caspase-8 in Human Leukemia Cells (Jurkat) by Dandelion Root Extract," *Journal of Ethnopharmacology* 133.1 (Jan 2011): 86–91. https://www.ncbi.nlm.nih.gov/pubmed/20849941 (accessed Apr 2018).

46. S. J. Chatterjee et al, "The Efficacy of Dandelion Root Extract in Inducing Apoptosis in Drug-Resistant Human Melanoma Cells," *Evidence-Based Complementary and Alternative Medicine* 2011 (Dec 2010): 129045. https://www.hindawi.com/journals/ecam/2011/129045/ (accessed Apr 2018).

47. Pamela Ovadje et al, "Selective Induction of Apoptosis and Autophagy Through Treatment with Dandelion Root Extract in Human Pancreatic Cancer Cells," *Pancreas* 41.7 (Oct 2012): 1039–47. https://www.ncbi.nlm.nih.gov/pubmed/22647733 (accessed Apr 2018).

48. Long-Gang Zhao et al, "Green Tea Consumption and Cause-Specific Mortality: Results from Two Prospective Cohort Studies in China," *Journal of Epidemiology* 27.1 (2017): 36–41. https://www.ncbi.nlm.nih.gov/pmc/articles/PMC5328738/ (accessed Apr 2018).

49. Gong Yang et al, "Green Tea Consumption and Colorectal Cancer Risk: A Report from the Shanghai Men's Health Study," *Carcinogenesis* 32.11 (Nov 2011): 1684–88. https://www.ncbi.nlm.nih.gov/pubmed/21856996 (accessed Apr 2018).

50. Hui-Hsuan Lin, Jing-Hsien Chen, and Chau-Jong Wang, "Chemopreventive Properties and Molecular Mechanisms of the Bioactive Compounds in Hibiscus Sabdariffa Linne," *Current Medicinal Chemistry* 18.8 (Feb 2011): 1245–54. https://www.researchgate.net/publication/49807880_Chemopreventive_Properties_and_Molecular_Mechanisms_of_the_Bioactive_Compounds_in_Hibiscus_Sabdariffa_Linne (accessed Apr 2018).

CHAPTER 9: Heroic Doses

1. Richard J. Bloomer et al, "A 21 Day Daniel Fast Improves Selected
    Biomarkers of Antioxidant Status and Oxidative Stress in Men and Women,"
    Nutrition and Metabolism 8.17 (Mar 2011). https://www.ncbi.nlm.nih.gov/
    pubmed/21414232 (accessed Apr 2018).

2. Dean Ornish et al, "Intensive Lifestyle Changes May Affect the Progression
    of Prostate Cancer," *The Journal of Urology* 174 (Sep 2005): 1065–70. https://
    www.ncbi.nlm.nih.gov/pubmed/16094059 (accessed Apr 2018).

3. G. A. Saxe, "Can Diet in Conjunction with Stress Reduction Affect the Rate
    of Increase in Prostate Specific Antigen after Biochemical Recurrence of
    Prostate Cancer?" *The Journal of Urology* 166.1 (Dec 2001): 2202–7. https://
    www.ncbi.nlm.nih.gov/pubmed/11696736 (accessed Apr 2018).

4. R. J. Barnard et al, "Effects of a Low-Fat, High-Fiber Diet and Exercise
    Program on Breast Cancer Risk Factors In Vivo and Tumor Cell Growth and
    Apoptosis In Vitro," *Nutrition and Cancer* 55.1 (Feb 2006): 28–34. https://
    www.ncbi.nlm.nih.gov/pubmed/16965238 (accessed Apr 2018).

5. Véronique Bouvard et al, "Carcinogenicity of Consumption of Red and
    Processed Meat," *The Lancet Oncology* 16.16 (Oct 2015): 1599–1600. http://
    www.thelancet.com/journals/lanonc/article/PIIS1470-2045(15)00444-1/
    abstract (accessed Apr 2018).

6. Giuseppe Lippi, Camilla Mattiuzzi, and Gianfranco Cervellin, "Meat
    Consumption and Cancer Risk: A Critical Review of Published Meta-
    Analyses," *ScienceDirect* 97 (Jan 2016): 1–14. https://www.ncbi.nlm.nih.gov/
    pubmed/26633248 (accessed Apr 2018); Jeanine M. Genkinger and Anita
    Koushik,"Meat Consumption and Cancer Risk" *PLoS Medicine* 4.12 (Dec
    2007): e345. https://www.ncbi.nlm.nih.gov/pmc/articles/PMC2121650
    (accessed May 2018).

7. R. J. Barnard et al, "Effects of a Low-Fat, High-Fiber Diet and Exercise
    Program on Breast Cancer Risk Factors In Vivo and Tumor Cell Growth and
    Apoptosis In Vitro," *Nutrition and Cancer* 55.1 (Feb 2006): 28–34. https://
    www.ncbi.nlm.nih.gov/pubmed/16965238 (accessed Apr 2018).

8. Barbara C. Halpern et al, "The Effect of Replacement of Methionine by
    Homocystine on Survival of Malignant and Normal Adult Mammalian Cells
    in Culture," *Proceedings of the National Academy of Sciences of the United States
    of America* 71.4 (Apr 1974): 1133–36. https://www.ncbi.nlm.nih.gov/pmc/
    articles/PMC388177/ (accessed Apr 2018).

9. Paul Cavuoto and Michael F. Fenech, "A Review of Methionine Dependency
    and the Role of Methionine Restriction in Cancer Growth Control and Life-
    Span Extension," *Cancer Treatment Reviews* 38.6 (Oct 2012): 726–36. https://
    www.ncbi.nlm.nih.gov/pubmed/22342103 (accessed Apr 2018).

Endnotes

10. I. Vucenik and A. M. Shamsuddin, "Protection Against Cancer by Dietary IP6 and Inositol," *Nutrition and Cancer* 55.2 (Feb 2006): 109–25. https://www.ncbi.nlm.nih.gov/pubmed/17044765 (accessed Apr 2018).

11. Morgan E. Levine, "Low Protein Intake Is Associated with a Major Reduction in IGF-1, Cancer, and Overall Mortality in the 65 and Younger but Not Older Population," *Cell Metabolism* 19.3 (Mar 2014): 407–17. https://www.ncbi.nlm.nih.gov/pubmed/24606898 (accessed Apr 2018).

12. Jae Jeng Yang et al, "Dietary Fat Intake and Lung Cancer Risk: A Pooled Analysis," *Journal of Clinical Oncology* 35.26 (Jul 2017): 3055–64. https://www.ncbi.nlm.nih.gov/pubmed/28742456 (accessed Apr 2018).

13. Semir Beyaz et al, "High Fat Diet Enhances Stemness and Tumorigenicity of Intestinal Progenitors," *Nature* 531.7592 (Mar 2016): 53–58. https://www.ncbi.nlm.nih.gov/pmc/articles/PMC4846772/ (accessed Apr 2018).

14. F. K. Tabung, S. E. Steck, and J. Zhang, "Dietary Inflammatory Index and Risk of Mortality: Findings from the Aerobics Center Longitudinal Study." Poster presented at American Institute for Cancer Research (AICR) Annual Research Conference, November 7, 2013, Bethesda, MD. https://www.ncbi.nlm.nih.gov/pubmed/24718872 (accessed Apr 2018).

15. Abina Sieri et al, "Dietary Fat Intake and Development of Specific Breast Cancer Subtypes," *Journal of the National Cancer Institute* 106.5 (Apr 2014): dju068. https://www.ncbi.nlm.nih.gov/pubmed/24718872 (accessed Apr 2018).

16. E. H. Allot et al, "Saturated Fat Intake and Prostate Cancer Aggressiveness: Results from the Population-Based North Carolina-Louisiana Prostate Cancer Project," *Prostate Cancer and Prostatic Diseases* 20 (Mar 2017): 48–54. https://www.ncbi.nlm.nih.gov/pubmed/27595916 (accessed Apr 2018).

17. Mary H. Ward, "Heme Iron from Meat and Risk of Adenocarcinoma of the Esophagus and Stomach," *European Journal of Cancer Prevention* 21.2 (Mar 2012): 134–38. https://www.ncbi.nlm.nih.gov/pmc/articles/PMC3261306/ (accessed Apr 2018).

18. Nadia M. Bastide, Fabrice H. F. Pierre, and Denis E. Corpet, "Heme Iron from Meat and Risk of Colorectal Cancer: A Meta-Analysis and a Review of the Mechanisms Involved," *Cancer Prevention Research* 4.2 (Feb 2011): 177–84. https://www.ncbi.nlm.nih.gov/pubmed/21209396 (accessed Apr 2018).

19. Nathalie M. Scheers et al, "Ferric Citrate and Ferric EDTA but Not Ferrous Sufate Drive Amphiregulin-Mediated Activation of the MAP Kinase ERK in Gut Epithelial Cancer Cells," *Oncotarget* 9 (Jul 2008): 996–1002. http://www.oncotarget.com/index.php?journal=oncotarget&page=article&op=view&path%5b%5d=24899 (accessed May 2018).

20. Leo R. Zacharski, "Decreased Cancer Risk after Iron Reduction in Patients with Peripheral Arterial Disease: Results from a Randomized Trial," *Journal of the National Cancer Institute* 100.14 (2018): 17066–17077. https://www.ncbi.nlm.nih.gov/pubmed/18612130 (accessed Apr 2018).

21. Dagfinn Aune et al, "Fruit and Vegetable Intake and the Risk of Cardiovascular Disease, Total Cancer and All-Cause Mortality—A Systematic Review and Dose-Response Meta-Analysis of Prospective Studies," *International Journal of Epidemiology* 46.3 (Jun 2017): 1029–56. https://www .ncbi.nlm.nih.gov/pubmed/28338764 (accessed Apr 2018).

22. Sarah Boseley, "Forget Five a Day, Eat 10 Portions of Fruit and Veg to Cut Risk of Early Death," *The Guardian* (Feb 2017). https://www.theguardian .com/society/2017/feb/23/five-day-10-portions-fruit-veg-cut-early-death (accessed Apr 2018).

23. S. De Flora, M. Bagnasco, and H. Vainio, "Modulation of Genotoxic and Related Effects by Carotenoids and Vitamin A in Experimental Models: Mechanistic Issues," *Mutagenesis* 14.2 (Mar 1999): 153–72. https://www.ncbi .nlm.nih.gov/pubmed/10229917 (accessed Apr 2018).

24. L. P. Christensen, "Aliphatic C(17)-Polyacetylenes of the Falcarinol Type as Potential Health Promoting Compounds in Food Plants of the Apiaceae Family," *Recent Patents on Food, Nutrition & Agriculture* 3.1 (Jan 2011): 64–77 . https://www.ncbi.nlm.nih.gov/pubmed/21114468 (accessed Apr 2018).

25. Ohio State University, "The Compound in the Mediterranean Diet That Makes Cancer Cells 'Mortal,'" *EurekAlert!* (May 2013). https://www.eurekalert .org/pub_releases/2013-05/osu-tci052013.php (accessed Apr 2018).

26. Rachel S. Rosenberg et al. "Modulation of Androgen and Progesterone Receptors by Phytochemicals in Breast Cancer Cell Lines," *Biochemical and Biophysical Research Communications* 248.3 (Aug 1998): 935–39. https://www .researchgate.net/publication/13581330_Modulation_of_Androgen_and_ Progesterone_Receptors_by_Phytochemicals_in_Breast_Cancer_Cell_Lines (accessed Apr 2018).

27. Xin Cai and Xuan Liu, "Inhibition of Thr-55 Phosphorylation Restores p53 Nuclear Localization and Sensitizes Cancer Cells to DNA Damage," *Proceedings of the National Academy of Sciences of the United States of America* 105.44 (Nov 2008): 16958–63. http://www.pnas.org/content/105/44/16958 (accessed Apr 2018).

28. M. Noroozi, W. J. Angerson, and M. E. Lean, "Effects of Flavonoids and Vitamin C on Oxidative DNA Damage to Human Lymphocytes," *The American Journal of Clinical Nutrition* 67.6 (Jun 1998): 1210–18. https://www .ncbi.nlm.nih.gov/pubmed/9625095 (accessed Apr 2018).

29. Theodore Fotsis et al, "Flavonoids, Dietary-Derived Inhibitors of Cell Proliferation and In Vitro Angiogenesis," *Cancer Research* 57.14 (Jul 1997): 2916–21. https://www.ncbi.nlm.nih.gov/pubmed/9230201 (accessed Apr 2018).

30. Hiroe Kikuzaki and Nobuji Nakatani, "Antioxidant Effects of Some Ginger Constituents," *Journal of Food Science* 58.6 (Nov 1993): 1407–10. https://www .researchgate.net/publication/227851087_Antioxidant_Effects_of_Some_ Ginger_Constituents (accessed Apr 2018).

Endnotes

31. H. Y. Zhou et al, "Experimental Study on Apoptosis Induced by Elemene in Glioma Cells," *Al Zheng* 22.9 (Sep 2003): 959–63. http://europepmc.org/abstract/med/12969529 (accessed Apr 2018).

32. Manjeshwar S. Baliga et al, "Update on the Chemopreventive Effects of Ginger and Its Phytochemicals," *Critical Reviews in Food Science and Nutrition* 51.6 (Jul 2011): 499–23 https://www.ncbi.nlm.nih.gov/pubmed/21929329 (accessed Apr 2018).

33. Magdalena Szejk, Joanna Kolodziejczyk-Czepas, and Halina Małgorzata Żbikowska, "Radioprotectors in Radiotherapy—Advances in the Potential Application of Phytochemicals," *Postepy Higieny* 70 (Jun 2016): 722–34. http://europepmc.org/abstract/med/27356603 (accessed Apr 2018).

34. Yue Zhou et al, "Dietary Natural Products for Prevention and Treatment of Liver Cancer," *Nutrients* 8.3 (Mar 2016): 156. https://www.ncbi.nlm.nih.gov/pmc/articles/PMC4808884/ (accessed Apr 2018).

35. Aesun Shin, Jeongseon Kim, and Sohee Park. "Gastric Cancer Epidemiology in Korea," *Journal of Gastric Cancer* 11.3 (Sep 2011): 135–40. https://www.ncbi.nlm.nih.gov/pmc/articles/PMC3204471/ (accessed Apr 2018).

36. Onica LeGendre, Paul A. S. Breslin, and David A. Foster, "(-)-Oleocanthal Rapidly and Selectively Induces Cancer Cell Death via Lysosomal Membrane Permeabilization," *Molecular & Cellular Oncology* 2.4 (Oct–Dec 015): e1006077. https://www.ncbi.nlm.nih.gov/pmc/articles/PMC4568762/ (accessed Apr 2018).

37. J. Gopal, "Authenticating Apple Cider Vinegar's Home Remedy Claims: Antibacterial, Antifungal, Antiviral Properties and Cytotoxicity Aspect," *National Product Research* 2017 (Dec 2017): 1–5. https://www.ncbi.nlm.nih.gov/pmc/articles/PMC4568762/ (accessed Apr 2018).

38. Anne Berit, C. Samuelsen, Jürgen Schrezenmeir, and Svein H. Knutsen, "Effects of Orally Administered Yeast-Derived Beta-glucans: A Review," *Molecular Nutrition and Food Research* 58.1 (Sep 2013): 183–93. https://onlinelibrary.wiley.com/doi/full/10.1002/mnfr.201300338 (accessed Apr 2018).

39. V. Vetvicka, B. P. Thornton, and G. D. Ross, "Targeting of Natural Killer Cells to Mammary Carcinoma via Naturally Occurring Tumor Cell-Bound iC3b and Beta-glucan-primed CR3 (CD11b/CD18)," *The Journal of Immunology* 159.2 (Jul 1997): 599–605. https://www.ncbi.nlm.nih.gov/pubmed/9218574 (accessed Apr 2018).

40. Gokhan Demir et al, "Beta glucan Induces Proliferation and Activation of Monocytes in Peripheral Blood of Patients with Advanced Breast Cancer," *International Immunopharmacology* 7.1 (Jan 2007): 113–16. https://www.ncbi.nlm.nih.gov/pubmed/17161824 (accessed Apr 2018).

41. Erdinc Yenidogan et al, "Effect of β-Glucan on Drain Fluid and Amount of Drainage Following Modified Radical Mastectomy," *Advances in Therapy*

31.1 (Jan 2014): 130–39. https://www.ncbi.nlm.nih.gov/pubmed/24421054 (accessed Apr 2018).

42. Soo Young Kim et al, "Biomedical Issues of Dietary Fiber β-Glucan," *Journal of Korean Medical Science* 21.5 (Oct 2006): 781–89. https://www.ncbi.nlm.nih .gov/pmc/articles/PMC2721983/ (accessed Apr 2018).

43. Temidayo Fadelu et al, "Nut Consumption and Survival in Patients with Stage III Colon Cancer: Results from CALGB 89803 (Alliance)," *Journal of Clinical Oncology* 36.11 (Apr 2018): 1112–1120. https://www.ncbi.nlm.nih .gov/pubmed/29489429 (accessed May 2018).

44. I. Garrido et al, "Polyphenols and Antioxidant Properties of Almond Skins: Influence of Industrial Processing," *Journal of Food Science* 3.2 (Mar 2008): C106–115. https://www.ncbi.nlm.nih.gov/pubmed/18298714 (accessed May 2018).

45. P. A. Brandt and L. J. Schouten, "Relationship of Tree Nut, Peanut and Peanut Butter Intake with Total and Cause-Specific Mortality: A Cohort Study and Meta-Analysis," *International Journal of Epidemiology* 44.3 (Jun 2015): 1038–1049. doi:10.1093/ije/dyv039 (accessed May 2018).

CHAPTER 10: Building a New Body

1. S. J. O'Keefe et al, "Rarity of Colon Cancer In Africans Is Associated with Low Animal Product Consumption, Not Fiber," *American Journal of Gastroenterology* 94.5 (May 1999): 1373–80. https://www.ncbi.nlm.nih.gov/ pubmed/10235221 (accessed Apr 2018).

2. Fernando P. Carvalho, João M. Oliveira, and Margarida Malta, "Radionuclides in Deep-Sea Fish and Other Organisms from the North Atlantic Ocean," *ICES Journal of Marine Science* 68.2 (Dec 2010): 333–40. https://www.researchgate .net/publication/273028830_Radionuclides_in_deep-sea_fish_and_other_ organisms_from_the_North_Atlantic_Ocean (accessed Apr 2018).

3. Alphonse Kelecom and Rita de Cássia dos Santos Gouvea, "Increase of Po–210 Levels in Human Semen Fluid After Mussel Ingestion," *Journal of Environmental Radioactivity* 102.5 (Feb 2011): 443–47. https://www .researchgate.net/publication/49812789_Increase_of_Po-210_levels_in_ human_semen_fluid_after_mussel_ingestion (accessed Apr 2018).

4. Daniel J. Madigan, Zofia Baumann, and Nicholas S. Fisher, "Pacific Bluefin Tuna Transport Fukushima-Derived Radionuclides from Japan to California," *Proceedings of the National Academy of Sciences of the United States of America* 109.24 (Jun 2012): 9483–86. https://www.ncbi.nlm.nih.gov/ pubmed/22645346 (accessed Apr 2018).

5. *Consumer Reports*, "Talking Turkey: Our New Tests Show Reasons for Concern," *Consumer Reports* (Jun 2013). https://www.consumerreports.org/ cro/magazine/2013/06/consumer-reports-investigation-talking-turkey/index .htm (accessed Apr 2018).

Endnotes

6. Food and Drug Administration, "2011 Retail Meat Report," *FDA* (2013). https://www.fda.gov/downloads/AnimalVeterinary/SafetyHealth/ AntimicrobialResistance/NationalAntimicrobialResistanceMonitoringSystem/ UCM334834.pdf (accessed Apr 2018).

7. Campaign on Human Health and Industrial Farming, "Record-High Antibiotic Sales for Meat and Poultry Production," *The PEW Charitable Trusts* (Feb 2013). http://www.pewtrusts.org/en/research-and-analysis/ analysis/2013/02/06/recordhigh-antibiotic-sales-for-meat-and-poultry -production (accessed Apr 2018).

8. Clett Erridge, "The Capacity of Foodstuffs to Induce Innate Immune Activation of Human Monocytes *In Vitro* Is Dependent on Food Content of Stimulants of Toll-Like Receptors 2 and 4," *British Journal of Nutrition* 105.1 (Jan 2011): 15–23. https://www.ncbi.nlm.nih.gov/pubmed/20849668 (accessed Apr 2018).

9. Rupali Deopurkar et al, "Differential Effects of Cream, Glucose, and Orange Juice on Inflammation, Endotoxin, and the Expression of Toll-Like Receptor-4 and Suppressor of Cytokine Signaling-3," *Diabetes Care* 33.5 (May 010): 991–97. https://www.ncbi.nlm.nih.gov/pmc/articles/PMC2858203/ (accessed Apr 2018).

10. C. R. Daniel et al, "Large Prospective Investigation of Meat Intake, Related Mutagens, and Risk of Renal Cell Carcinoma," *The American Journal of Clinical Nutrition* 95.1 (Jan 2012): 155–162. https://www.ncbi.nlm.nih.gov/ pubmed/22170360 (accessed May 2018).

11. J. Wang et al, "Carcinogen Metabolism Genes, Red Meat and Poultry Intake, and Colorectal Cancer Risk," *International Journal of Cancer* 130.8 (Apr 2012): 1898–1907. https://www.ncbi.nlm.nih.gov/pubmed/21618522 (accessed May 2018).

12. E. de Stefani et al, "Meat Consumption, Meat Cooking and Risk of Lung Cancer Among Uruguayan Men," *Asian Pacific Journal of Cancer Prevention* 11.6 (2010): 1713–1717. https://www.ncbi.nlm.nih.gov/pubmed/21338220 (accessed May 2018).

13. Esther M. John et al, "Meat Consumption, Cooking Practices, Meat Mutagens and Risk of Prostate Cancer," *Nutrition and Cancer* 63.4 (2011): 525–537. https://www.ncbi.nlm.nih.gov/pmc/articles/PMC3516139 (accessed May 2018).

14. K. E. Anderson et al, "Pancreatic Cancer Risk: Associations with Meat-Derived Carcinogen Intake in the Prostate, Lung, Colorectal, and Ovarian Cancer Screening Trial (PLCO) Cohort," *Molecular Carcinogenesis* 51.1 (Jan 2012): 128–137. https://www.ncbi.nlm.nih.gov/pubmed/22162237 (accessed May 2018).

15. Donghui Li et al, "Dietary Mutagen Exposure and Risk of Pancreatic Cancer," *Cancer Epidemiology, Biomarkers & Prevention* 16.4 (Apr 2007): 655–661. https://www.ncbi.nlm.nih.gov/pubmed/17416754 (accessed May 2018).

16. K. Puangsombat et al, "Occurrence of Heterocyclic Amines in Cooked Meat Products," *Meat Science* 90.3 (Mar 2012): 739–746. https://www.ncbi.nlm.nih .gov/pubmed/22129588 (accessed May 2018).

17. Ola Viegas et al, "Inhibitory Effect of Antioxidant-Rich Marinades on the Formation of Heterocyclic Aromatic Amines in Pan-Fried Beef," *Journal of Agricultural and Food Chemistry* 60.24 (Jun 2012): 6235–40. https://www.ncbi .nlm.nih.gov/pubmed/22642699 (accessed Apr 2018).

18. J. S. Smith, F. Ameri, and P. Gadgil, "Effect of Marinades on the Formation of Heterocyclic Amines in Grilled Beef Steaks," *Journal of Food Science* 73.6 (2008): 100–105. https://www.ncbi.nlm.nih.gov/pubmed/19241593 (accessed Apr 2018).

19. Afsaneh Farhadian et al, "Effects of Marinating on the Formation of Polycyclic Aromatic Hydrocarbons (Benzo[a]pyrene, Benzo[b]uoranthene and Fluoranthene) in Grilled Beef Meat," *Food Control* 28.2 (Dec 2012): 420–25. https://www.researchgate.net/publication/257398846_Effects_ of_marinating_on_the_formation_of_polycyclic_aromatic_hydrocarbons_ benzoapyrene_benzobfluoranthene_and_fluoranthene_in_grilled_beef_meat (accessed Apr 2018).

20. Timothy J. Key et al, "Cancer Incidence in Vegetarians: Results from the European Prospective Investigation into Cancer and Nutrition," *The American Journal of Clinical Nutrition* 89.5 (May 2009): 1620–26. https://www .ncbi.nlm.nih.gov/pubmed/19279082 (accessed Apr 2018).

CHAPTER 11: Take Out the Trash

1. Hyun-Wook Lee et al, "E-cigarette Smoke Damages DNA and Reduces Repair Activity in Mouse Lung, Heart, and Bladder as well as in Human Lung and Bladder Cells," *Proceedings of the National Academy of Sciences of the United States of America* (Jan 2018). http://www.pnas.org/content/ early/2018/01/25/1718185115 (accessed Apr 2018).

2. Anthony Samsel and Stephanie Seneff, "Glyphosate's Suppression of Cytochrome P450 Enzymes and Amino Acid Biosynthesis by the Gut Microbiome: Pathways to Modern Diseases," *Entropy* 15.4 (Apr 2013): 1416– 63. http://www.mdpi.com/1099-4300/15/4/1416 (accessed Apr 2018).

3. Siriporn Thongprakaisang et al, "Glyphosate Induces Human Breast Cancer Cells Growth via Estrogen Receptors," *Food and Chemical Toxicology* 59 (Jun 2013): 129–36. https://www.researchgate.net/publication/237146763_ Glyphosate_induces_human_breast_cancer_cells_growth_via_estrogen_ receptors (accessed Apr 2018).

4. Carey Gillam, "Weedkiller Found in Granola and Crackers, Internal FDA Emails Show," *The Guardian* (Apr 2018). https://www.theguardian.com/ us-news/2018/apr/30/fda-weedkiller-glyphosate-in-food-internal-emails (accessed May 2018).

Endnotes

5. Liza Oates et al, "Reduction in Urinary Organophosphate Pesticide Metabolites in Adults After a Week-Long Organic Diet," *Journal of Environmental Research* 132 (Jun 2014): 105–11. https://www.ncbi.nlm.nih.gov/pubmed/24769399 (accessed Apr 2018).

6. Asa Bradman et al, "Effect of Organic Diet Intervention on Pesticide Exposures in Young Children Living in Low-Income Urban and Agricultural Communities," *Environmental Health Perspectives* 123.10 (Oct 2015): 1086–93. https://www.ncbi.nlm.nih.gov/pubmed/25861095 (accessed Apr 2018).

7. Zhi-Yong Yang et al, "Effects of Home Preparation on Pesticide Residues in Cabbage," *Food Control* 18.12 (Dec 2007): 1484–1487. https://www.sciencedirect.com/science/article/pii/S0956713506002696 (accessed May 2018).

8. "Citizen Petition in re: Use of Hydrofluorosilic Acid in Drinking Water Systems of the United States," *EPA* (Apr 2013). https://www.epa.gov/sites/production/files/documents/tsca_21_petition_hfsa_2013-04-22.pdf (accessed May 2018).

9. Sherri A. Mason, Victoria Welch, and Joseph Neratko, "Synthetic Polymer Contamination in Bottled Water," *Fredonia* (2018). https://orbmedia.org/sites/default/files/FinalBottledWaterReport.pdf (accessed Apr 2018).

10. R. Vogt et al, "Cancer and Non-Cancer Health Effects from Food Contaminant Exposures for Children and Adults in California: A Risk Assessment," *Environmental Health* 11 (Nov 2012): 83. https://www.ncbi.nlm.nih.gov/pubmed/23140444 (accessed May 2018).

11. Chris Exley, "Strong Evidence Linking Aluminum and Alzheimer's," *Hippocratic Post* (Dec 2016). https://www.hippocraticpost.com/mental-health/strong-evidence-linking-aluminium-alzheimers/ (accessed Apr 2018).

12. Mike Adams, "Natural Consumer Products Found Contaminated with Cancer-Causing 1,4-Dioxane in Groundbreaking Analysis Released by OCA," *Organic Consumers Association* (Mar 2008). https://www.organicconsumers.org/news/natural-consumer-products-found-contaminated-cancer-causing-14-dioxane-groundbreaking-analysis (accessed Apr 2018).

13. P. D. Darbre, "Aluminium, Antiperspirants and Breast Cancer," *Journal of Inorganic Biochemistry* 99.9 (Sep 2005): 1912–19. https://www.ncbi.nlm.nih.gov/pubmed/16045991 (accessed Apr 2018).

14. G. M. Richardson et al, "Mercury Exposure and Risks from Dental Amalgam in the US Population, Post-2000," *Science of the Total Environment* 409.20 (Sep 2011): 4257–68. https://www.ncbi.nlm.nih.gov/pubmed/21782213 (accessed Apr 2018).

15. José G. Dórea et al, "Speciation of Methyl- and Ethyl-Mercury in Hair of Breastfed Infants Acutely Exposed to Thimerosal-Containing Vaccines," *Clinica Chimica Acta* 412.17–18 (Aug 2011): 1563–66. https://www.ncbi.nlm.nih.gov/pubmed/21782213 (accessed Apr 2018).

16. Brian C. McDonald et al, "Volatile Chemical Products Emerging as Largest Petrochemical Source of Urban Organic Emissions," *Science* 359.6377 (Feb 2018): 760–64. http://science.sciencemag.org/content/359/6377/760 (accessed Apr 2018).

17. The American Cancer Society medical and editorial content team, "Radon and Cancer," *The American Cancer Society* (Sep 2015). https://www.cancer.org/cancer/cancer-causes/radiation-exposure/radon.html (accessed Apr 2018).

18. Wikipedia contributors, "NASA Clean Air Study," *Wikipedia, The Free Encyclopedia* (Jan 2018). https://en.wikipedia.org/w/index.php?title=NASA_Clean_Air_Study&oldid=821719488 (accessed Jan 2018).

19. B. C. Wolverton, Rebecca C. McDonald, and E. A. Watkins Jr., "Foliage Plants for Removing Indoor Air Pollutants from Energy-Efficient Homes," *JSTOR*, 38.2 (Apr–Jun 1984): 224–28. https://www.jstor.org/stable/4254614 (accessed Apr 2018).

20. Orianne Dumas et al, "Occupational Exposure to Disinfectants and Asthma Control in US Nurses," *European Respiratory Journal* 50.4 (Oct 2017): 700237. https://www.ncbi.nlm.nih.gov/pubmed/28982772 (accessed Apr 2018). "Occupational exposure to disinfectants and COPD incidence in US nurses: a prospective cohort study," The air indoor pollution session, 08.30–0.30 hours CEST, Monday 11 September, Brown 1+2 (south).

21. Øistein Svanes et al, "Cleaning at Home and at Work in Relation to Lung Function Decline and Airway Obstruction," *American Journal of Respiratory and Critical Care Medicine* (2018). http://www.thoracic.org/about/newsroom/press-releases/resources/women-cleaners-lung-function.pdf (accessed Apr 2018).

22. University of Washington, "Scented Laundry Products Emit Hazardous Chemicals Through Dryer Vents," *EurekAlert!* (Aug 2011). https://www.eurekalert.org/pub_releases/2011-08/uow-slp082311.php (accessed Apr 2018).

23. Euro Pukkala et al, "Occupation and Cancer—Follow-up of 15 Million People in Five Nordic Countries," *Acta Oncologica* 48.5 (2009): 646–90. https://www.ncbi.nlm.nih.gov/pubmed/19925375 (accessed Apr 2018).

24. Andrea't Mannetje, Amanda Eng, and Neil Pearce, "Farming, Growing Up on a Farm, and Haematological Cancer Mortality," *Occupational & Environmental Medicine* 69.2 (Feb 2012): 126–32. https://www.ncbi.nlm.nih.gov/pubmed/2179574 (accessed Apr 2018).

25. Gregory J. Tranah, Paige M. Bracci, and Elizabeth A. Holly, "Domestic and Farm-Animal Exposures and Risk of Non-Hodgkin Lymphoma in a Population-Based Study in the San Francisco Bay Area," *Cancer Epidemiological, Biomarkers & Preventions* 17.9 (Sep 2008): 2382–87. https://www.ncbi.nlm.nih.gov/pmc/articles/PMC2946322/ (accessed Apr 2018).

26. Samuel Milham, "Historical Evidence That Electrification Caused the 20th Century Epidemic of 'Diseases of Civilization,'" *Medical Hypotheses* 74.2 (Feb

2010): 337–45. http://www.sammilham.com/historical%20evidence.pdf (accessed Apr 2018).

27. N. Wertheimer and E. Leeper, "Electrical Wiring Configurations and Childhood Cancer," *American Journal of Epidemiology* 109.3 (Mar 1979): 273–84. https://www.ncbi.nlm.nih.gov/pubmed/453167 (accessed Apr 2018).

28. Martin L. Pall, "Wi-Fi Is an Important Threat to Human Health," *Environmental Research* 164 (Jul 2018): 405–416. https://www.sciencedirect.com/science/article/pii/S0013935118300355?via=ihub (accessed May 2018).

29. Ali H. Mokdad et al, "Trends and Patterns of Disparities in Cancer Mortality Among US Counties, 1980–2014," *JAMA* 317.4 (Jan 2017): 388–406. https://www.ncbi.nlm.nih.gov/pmc/articles/PMC5617139/ (accessed Apr 2018).

30. "Cancer Stat Facts: Brain and Other Nervous System," *National Cancer Institute: Surveillance, Epidemiology, and End Results Program.* https://seer.cancer.gov/statfacts/html/brain.html (accessed May 2018).

31. Alasdair Philips et al, "Brain Tumours: Rise in Glioblastoma Multiforme Incidence in England 1995–2015 Suggests an Adverse Environmental or Lifestyle Factor," *Journal of Environmental and Public Health* (May 2018). https://www.hindawi.com/journals/jeph/aip/7910754/ (accessed May 2018).

32. Suzanne Wu, "Fasting Triggers Stem Cell Regeneration of Damaged, Old Immune System," *USC News* (Jun 2014). https://news.usc.edu/63669/fasting-triggers-stem-cell-regeneration-of-damaged-old-immune-system/ (accessed Apr 2018).

33. C. Lee et al, "Fasting Cycles Retard Growth of Tumors and Sensitize a Range of Cancer Cell Types to Chemotherapy," *Science Translational Medicine* 4.124 (Mar 2012): 124ra27. https://www.ncbi.nlm.nih.gov/pmc/articles/PMC3608686/ (accessed Apr 2018).

34. Tanya B. Dorff et al, "Safety and Feasibility of Fasting in Combination with Platinum-Based Chemotherapy," *BMC Cancer* 16.360 (Jun 2016): 1–9. https://bmccancer.biomedcentral.com/articles/10.1186/s12885-016-2370-6 (accessed Apr 2018).

35. Min Wei et al, "Fasting-Mimicking Diet and Markers/Risk Factors for Aging, Diabetes, Cancer, and Cardiovascular Disease," *Science Translational Medicine* 9.377 (Feb 2017): eaai8700. https://www.ncbi.nlm.nih.gov/pubmed/28202779 (accessed Apr 2018).

CHAPTER 12: Let's Get Physical

1. Frank W. Booth, Christian K. Roberts, and Matthew J. Laye, "Lack of Exercise Is a Major Cause of Chronic Diseases," *Comprehensive Physiology* 2.2 (Jan 2012): 1143–211. https://www.ncbi.nlm.nih.gov/pmc/articles/PMC4241367/ (accessed Apr 2018).

2. National Cancer Institute, "Physical Activity and Cancer," *NIH* (Jan 2017). https://www.cancer.gov/about-cancer/causes-prevention/risk/obesity/physical-activity-fact-sheet (accessed Apr 2018).

3. L. Packer, "Oxidants, Antioxidant Nutrients and the Athlete," *Journal of Sports Science* 15.3 (Jun 1997): 353–63. https://www.ncbi.nlm.nih.gov/pubmed/9232561 (accessed Apr 2018).

4. Jake Emmett, "The Physiology of Marathon Running," *Marathon and Beyond* (2007). http://www.marathonandbeyond.com/choices/emmett.htm (accessed Apr 2018).

5. Roy J. Shephard and Pang N. Shek, "Potential Impact of Physical Activity and Sport on the Immune System—a Brief Review," *British Journal of Sports Medicine* 28.4 (Dec 1994): 247–55. https://www.ncbi.nlm.nih.gov/pubmed/7894956 (accessed Apr 2018).

6. Brett R. Gordon et al, "The Effects of Resistance Exercise Training on Anxiety: A Meta-Analysis and Meta-Regression Analysis of Randomized Controlled Trials," *Sports Medicine* 47.12 (Aug 2017): 2521–32. https://www.researchgate.net/publication/318102093_The_Effect_of_Resistance_Exercise_Training_on_Anxiety_Symptoms_A_Systematic_Review_and_Meta-Analysis (accessed Apr 2018).

7. R. Barrès et al, "Acute Exercise Remodels Promoter Methylation in Human Skeletal Muscle," *Cell Metabolism* 15.3 (Mar 2012): 405–11. https://www.ncbi.nlm.nih.gov/pubmed/22405075 (accessed Apr 2018).

8. Urho M. Kujala, "Relationship of Leisure-Time Physical Activity and Mortality: The Finnish Twin Cohort," *JAMA* 279.6 (Feb 1998): 440–44. https://www.ncbi.nlm.nih.gov/pubmed/9466636 (accessed Apr 2018).

9. John P. Pierce, "Greater Survival After Breast Cancer in Physically Active Women with High Vegetable-Fruit Intake Regardless of Obesity," *Journal of Clinical Oncology* 25.17 (Jun 2007): 2345–51. https://www.ncbi.nlm.nih.gov/pmc/articles/PMC2274898/ (accessed Apr 2018).

10. Christine Dethlefsen, "Exercise-Induced Catecholamines Activate the Hippo Tumor Suppressor Pathway to Reduce Risks of Breast Cancer Development," *Cancer Research* 77.18 (Sep 2017): 4894–904. http://cancerres.aacrjournals.org/content/early/2017/09/07/0008-5472.CAN-16-3125 (accessed Apr 2018).

11. Carlos A. Celis-Morales et al, "Association Between Active Commuting and Incident Cardiovascular Disease, Cancer, and Mortality: Prospective Cohort Study," *BMJ* 357 (Apr 2017): j1456. https://www.bmj.com/content/357/bmj.j1456 (accessed Apr 2018).

12. Stephanie E. Bonn et al, "Physical Activity and Survival Among Men Diagnosed with Prostate Cancer," *Cancer Epidemiology, Biomarkers & Prevention* 24.1 (Dec 2014): 57–64. http://cebp.aacrjournals.org/content/early/2014/11/26/1055-9965.EPI-14-0707 (accessed Apr 2018).

Endnotes

13. Hannah Arem et al, "Pre- and Postdiagnosis Physical Activity, Television Viewing, and Mortality Among Patients with Colorectal Cancer in the National Institutes of Health–AARP Diet and Health Study," *Journal of Clinical Oncology* 33.2 (Jan 2015): 180–88. https://www.ncbi.nlm.nih.gov/ pmc/articles/PMC4279238/ (accessed Apr 2018).

14. Erin J. Howden et al, "Reversing the Cardiac Effects of Sedentary Aging in Middle Age—a Randomized Controlled Trial: Implications for Heart Failure Prevention," *Circulation* 137.14 (Jan 2018): 1–18. http://circ.ahajournals.org/ content/early/2018/01/03/CIRCULATIONAHA.117.030617 (accessed Apr 2018).

15. Niharika Arora Duggal, "Major Features of Immunesenescence, Including Reduced Thymic Output, Are Ameliorated by High Levels of Physical Activity in Adulthood," *Aging Cell* 17.2 (Mar 2018): e12750. https://onlinelibrary .wiley.com/doi/full/10.1111/acel.12750 (accessed Apr 2018).

16. Margaret E. Sears, Kathleen J. Kerr, and Riina I. Bray, "Arsenic, Cadmium, Lead, and Mercury in Sweat: A Systematic Review," *Journal of Environmental and Public Health* 2012 (2012): 1–10. https://www.hindawi.com/journals/ jeph/2012/184745/ (accessed Apr 2018).

17. H. G. Ainsleigh, "Beneficial Effects of Sun Exposure on Cancer Mortality," *Preventative Medicine* 22.1 (Jan 1993): 132–40. https://www.ncbi.nlm.nih.gov/ pubmed/8475009 (accessed Apr 2018).

18. James L. Oschman, Gaétan Chevalier, and Richard Brown, "The Effects of Grounding (Earthing) on Inflammation, the Immune Response, Wound Healing, and Prevention and Treatment of Chronic Inflammatory and Autoimmune Diseases," *Journal of Inflammation Research* 8 (Mar 2015): 83–96. https://www.ncbi.nlm.nih.gov/pmc/articles/PMC4378297/ (accessed Apr 2018).

19. Q. Li et al, "Forest Bathing Enhances Human Natural Killer Activity and Expression of Anti-Cancer Proteins," *International Journal of Immunopathology and Pharmacology* 20.2 (Apr–Jun 2007): 3–8. https://www.ncbi.nlm.nih.gov/ pubmed/17903349 (accessed Apr 2018).

20. Q. Li et al, "Acute Effects of Walking in Forest Environments on Cardiovascu-lar and Metabolic Parameters," *European Journal of Applied Physiology* 111.11 (Nov 2011): 2845–53. https://www.ncbi.nlm.nih.gov/pubmed/21431424 (accessed Apr 2018).

21. Q. Li et al, "Effect of Phytoncide from Trees on Human Natural Killer Cell Function," *International Journal of Immunopathology and Pharmacology* 22.4 (Oct –Dec 2009): 951–59. https://www.ncbi.nlm.nih.gov/pubmed/20074458 (accessed Apr 2018).

22. Centers for Disease Control and Prevention, "1 in 3 Adults Don't Get Enough Sleep," *CDC* (reviewed Feb 2016). https://www.cdc.gov/media/ releases/2016/p0215-enough-sleep.html (accessed Apr 2018).

23. Sheldon Cohen et al, "Sleep Habits and Susceptibility to the Common Cold," *Archives of Internal Medicine* 169.1 (Jan 2009): 62–67. https://www.ncbi.nlm .nih.gov/pmc/articles/PMC2629403/ (accessed Apr 2018).

24. Kenneth P. Wright, Jr. et al, "Entrainment of the Human Circadian Clock to the Natural Light-Dark Cycle," *Current Biology* 23.16 (Aug 2013): 1554–58. https://www.ncbi.nlm.nih.gov/pubmed/23910656 (accessed Apr 2018)

25. Ya Li et al, "Melatonin for the Prevention and Treatment of Cancer," *Oncotarget* 8.24 (Jun 2017): 39896–921. https://www.ncbi.nlm.nih.gov/pmc/ articles/PMC5503661/ (accessed Apr 2018).

26. M. Sánchez-Hidalgo et al, "Melatonin, a Natural Programmed Cell Death Inducer in Cancer," *Current Medicinal Chemistry* 19.22 (2012): 3805–21. https://www.ncbi.nlm.nih.gov/pubmed/22612707 (accessed Apr 2018).

27. Mariangela Rondanelli et al, "Update on the Role of Melatonin in the Prevention of Cancer Tumorigenesis and in the Management of Cancer Correlates, Such as Sleep-Wake and Mood Disturbances: Review and Remarks," *Aging Clinical and Experimental Research* 25.5 (Oct 2013): 499–510. https://www.ncbi.nlm.nih.gov/pubmed/24046037 (accessed Apr 2018).

28. Joshua J. Gooley et al, "Exposure to Room Light before Bedtime Suppresses Melatonin Onset and Shortens Melatonin Duration in Humans," *The Journal of Clinical Endocrinology & Metabolism* 96.3 (Mar 2011): E463–72. https:// academic.oup.com/jcem/article/96/3/E463/2597236 (accessed Apr 2018).

29. Shadab A. Rahman et al, "Circadian Phase Resetting by a Single Short-Duration Light Exposure," *JCI Insight* 2.7 (Apr 2017): e89494. https://www .ncbi.nlm.nih.gov/pmc/articles/PMC5374060 (accessed May 2018).

30. Eva S. Schernhammer and Susan E. Hankinson, "Urinary Melatonin Levels and Postmenopausal Breast Cancer Risk in the Nurses' Health Study Cohort," *Cancer Epidemiology, Biomarkers and Prevention* 18.1 (Jan 2009): 74–79. https:// www.ncbi.nlm.nih.gov/pmc/articles/PMC3036562/ (accessed Apr 2018).

31. Harvard Medical School, "Blue Light Has a Dark Side," *Harvard Health Publishing* (May 2012). https://www.health.harvard.edu/staying-healthy/ blue-light-has-a-dark-side (accessed Apr 2018).

32. Ariadna Garcia-Saenz et al, "Evaluating the Association between Artificial Light-at-Night Exposure and Breast and Prostate Cancer Risk in Spain (MCC-Spain Study)," *Environmental Health Perspectives* 126.4 (Apr 2018). https:// ehp.niehs.nih.gov/ehp1837 (accessed May 2018).

33. Alina Bradford, "How Blue LEDs Affect Sleep," *Live Science* (Feb 2016). https://www.livescience.com/53874-blue-light-sleep.html (accessed Apr 2018).

34. J. Kliukiene, T. Tynes, and A. Andersen, "Risk of Breast Cancer Among Norwegian Women with Visual Impairment," *British Journal of Cancer* 84.3 (Feb 2001): 397–99. https://www.ncbi.nlm.nih.gov/pmc/articles/ PMC2363754/ (accessed Apr 2018).

Endnotes

35. "Melatonin Drug Interactions," *Drugs.com* (updated Mar 2018). https://www.drugs.com/drug-interactions/melatonin.html (accessed Apr 2018).

36. Ye-min Wang et al,"The Efficacy and Safety of Melatonin in Concurrent Chemotherapy or Radiotherapy for Solid Tumors: A Meta-Analysis of Randomized Controlled Trials," *Cancer Chemotherapy and Pharmacology* 69.5 (May 2012): 1213–20. https://www.ncbi.nlm.nih.gov/pubmed/22271210 (accessed Apr 2018).

37. Jane Brody, "Cheating Ourselves of Sleep," *New York Times* (Jun 2013). https://well.blogs.nytimes.com/2013/06/17/cheating-ourselves-of-sleep/ (accessed Apr 2018).

38. Cheryl L. Thompson et al, "Short Duration of Sleep Increases Risk of Colorectal Adenoma,"" *Cancer* 117.4 (Feb 2011): 841–47. https://www.ncbi.nlm.nih.gov/pmc/articles/PMC3021092/ (accessed Apr 2018).

39. Claudia Trudel-Fitzgerald et al, "Sleep and Survival Among Women with Breast Cancer: 30 Years of Follow-up within the Nurses' Health Study," *British Journal of Cancer* 116 (Apr 2017): 1239–46. https://www.ncbi.nlm.nih.gov/pubmed/28359077 (accessed Apr 2018).

40. Dave Levitan, "Longer Sleep Linked to Increased Mortality Risk in Breast Cancer," *Cancer Network* (Apr 2017). http://www.cancernetwork.com/breast-cancer/longer-sleep-linked-increased-mortality-risk-breast-cancer (accessed Apr 2018).

41. Fahed Hakim et al, "Fragmented Sleep Accelerates Tumor Growth and Progression Through Recruitment of Tumor-Associated Macrophages and TLR4 Signaling," *Cancer Research* 74.5 (Mar 2014): 1329–37. https://www.ncbi.nlm.nih.gov/pmc/articles/PMC4247537/ (accessed Apr 2018).

42. Daniel F. Kripke, "Hypnotic Drug Risks of Mortality, Infection, Depression, and Cancer: But Lack of Benefit," *F1000Research* 5 (May 2016): 918. https://www.ncbi.nlm.nih.gov/pmc/articles/PMC4890308/ (accessed Apr 2018).

43. Lisa M. Wu et al, "The Effect of Systematic Light Exposure on Sleep in a Mixed Group of Fatigued Cancer Survivors," *Journal of Clinical Sleep Medicine* 14.1 (Jan 2017): 31–39. https://www.ncbi.nlm.nih.gov/pmc/articles/PMC5734890/ (accessed Apr 2018).

44. Lisa Rapaport, "Bright Light Therapy May Help Fatigued Cancer Survivors Sleep Better," *Reuters* (2017). https://www.reuters.com/article/us-health-cancer-sleep/bright-light-therapy-may-help-fatigued-cancer-survivors-sleep-better-idUSKBN1FF2QY (accessed Apr 2018).

45. U.S. Department of Health and Human Services, "How Sleep Clears the Brain," *NIH* (Oct 2013). https://www.nih.gov/news-events/nih-research-matters/how-sleep-clears-brain (accessed Apr 2018).

46. Catherine R. Marinac et al, "Prolonged Nightly Fasting and Breast Cancer Prognosis," *JAMA Oncology* 2.8 (Aug 2016): 1049–55. https://www.ncbi.nlm.nih.gov/pmc/articles/PMC4982776/ (accessed Apr 2018).

CHAPTER 13: Under Pressure

1. Sazzad Hassan et al, "Behavioral Stress Accelerates Prostate Cancer Development in Mice," *The Journal of Clinical Investigation* 123.2 (Feb 2013): 874–86. https://www.ncbi.nlm.nih.gov/pmc/articles/PMC3561807/ (accessed Apr 2018).

2. Caroline P. Le et al, "Chronic Stress in Mice Remodels Lymph Vasculature to Promote Tumour Cell Dissemination," *Nature Communications* 7 (Mar 2016): 10634. https://www.ncbi.nlm.nih.gov/pmc/articles/PMC4773495/ (accessed Apr 2018).

3. Alice Donaldson, "Stress Can Allow Cancer to Spread Faster Through the Body, New Research on Mice Shows," *ABC News* (Jun 2016). http://www.abc.net.au/news/2016-06-28/stress-can-speed-up-spread-of-cancer-in-body-scientists-say/7548024 (accessed Apr 2018).

4. Ohio State University, "The Stress and Cancer Link: 'Master-Switch' Stress Gene Enables Cancer's Spread," *ScienceDaily* (Aug 2013). www.sciencedaily.com/releases/2013/08/130822194143.htm (accessed Apr 2018).

5. L. S. Berk et al, "Modulation of Neuroimmune Parameters During the Eustress of Humor-Associated Mirthful Laughter," *Alternative Therapies in Health and Medicine* 7.2 (Mar 2001): 62–72, 74–76. https://www.ncbi.nlm.nih.gov/pubmed/11253418 (accessed May 2018).

6. Daisy Fancourt et al, "Singing Modulates Mood, Stress, Cortisol, Cytokine and Neuropeptide Activity in Cancer Patients and Carers," *Ecancermedicalscience* 10 (Apr 2016): 631. https://www.ncbi.nlm.nih.gov/pmc/articles/PMC4854222/ (accessed Apr 2018).

CHAPTER 14: Spiritual Healing

1. W. A. Brown, "Expectation, the Placebo Effect and the Response to Treatment," *Rhode Island Medical Journal* 98.5 (May 2015): 19–21. https://www.ncbi.nlm.nih.gov/pubmed/25938400 (accessed May 2018).

2. K. Wartolowska et al, "Use of Placebo Controls in the Evaluation of Surgery: Systematic Review," *BMJ* 348 (May 2014): g3253. https://www.ncbi.nlm.nih.gov/pubmed/24850821 (accessed May 2018).

INDEX

Index

ACKNOWLEDGMENTS

THIS BOOK TOOK ME MANY YEARS, much longer than it should have, because I am an excellent procrastinator and prefer sprints over marathons. A finished book might be my biggest miracle of all.

Thank you to all of the amazing death-defying cancer survivors, integrative medical doctors, and holistic healers I have ever interviewed. You have taught me so much about health and healing and you inspire me every day.

While writing this book, before I had an agent (still don't) or a publisher, I had a dream, a vision, a premonition, a prophecy—I don't know what to call it—that I would not have to play the traditional publishing game, i.e., convincing an agent to represent me and convincing a publisher to publish my book. I sensed that the perfect publisher would come to me at the perfect time. And that is exactly what happened. Thank you Liana Werner-Gray. You were instrumental in that perfect timing.

Thank you to Perry Wilson for introducing me to Howie Klausner. Thank you to Howie for introducing me to Matt West. Thank you to Matt West, for taking my sprawling mess of a manuscript, dissecting it piece by piece, and helping me develop it into something that actually resembled a book. You saw the forest for the trees. You have an amazing gift, my brother.

To my Hay House Family. Thank you to Reid Tracy and Patty Gift at Hay House for believing in me and my message and for publishing this book! Thank you to my editor, Lisa Cheng, for your enthusiastic support and gracious encouragement in the refinement process. And to everyone else at Hay House—thank you for all the work you did behind the scenes to bring this baby to life.

Thank you to Rev. George Malkmus, Dr. Richard Schulze, Dr. Lorraine Day, Anne and David Frahm, Dr. Hulda Clark, and Dr. Max Gerson. Your books and tapes were all I had in the beginning, and they gave me the courage to step out into the unknown and start my healing adventure. I stand on your shoulders. Thank you to John Smothers and the late Roy Page, M.D., your support meant the world to me in my darkest hour.

Thank you to Dr. Michael Greger at nutritionfacts.org. Your commitment to bring evidence-based nutritional science to the masses has had a profound impact on my life and my work, including the content of this book, and is changing the world.

To my dear friends in the health and wellness world who have helped me reach more people, Ty and Charlene Bollinger, Kevin Gianni, Robyn Openshaw, Dr. Eric Zielinski, John Robbins, Ocean Robbins, Dr. Kelly Turner, James Colquhoun, and so many others—thank you.

To Mark Rogers, I am grateful for your friendship and partnership in helping me share the SQUARE ONE Program with hundreds of thousands of people around the world. If we ever meet in person, it's going to be weird for me.

To my family, Mom and Dad, David and Catharine Wark, for loving me unconditionally, always supporting me, and believing in me when I didn't believe in myself. To my sister, Lindsay Bean, and my drummer/brother-in-law/best man Brad Bean, and to my wonderful in-laws, Ernie and Lynn, Kathy, Donna, Ashley and Josh, Beth and Jeremy, David and Liza, Meredith and Alan, Rob, Melody, Lucas, Meryl, and all of your significant others, thank you for graciously adopting me into your big fun family. Thank you for your prayers. I love you all so much. Aunt Connie, you are dearly missed.

Acknowledgments

To my beautiful and brilliant daughters, Marin and Mackenzie, you bring me so much joy. I am so proud of you both. I am blessed beyond words to be your dad and to be alive to watch you grow up. You make me a rich man.

And to the love of my life, my dream girl and wonderful wife, Micah. Twenty-two years and counting! Thank you for loving me, accepting me for who I am, sticking with me when I was sick and broke, and for putting up with me and all my crazy health obsessions over the years. See, it was worth it! We've weathered the storm and created an amazing life and family together. I love you with all my heart, and I can't imagine life without you. Let's grow old together and die at the same time.

And finally, a massive thank-you to you, my friends, fans, followers, and readers. Without your support, I would have not been able to sustain this mission. I measure my success not by the number of dollars I make, or the number of books I sell, but by the number of people I'm able to encourage, inspire, inform, empower, and ultimately save. You all have been instrumental in my success. Thank you for helping me spread the message of hope—that cancer can be healed.

ABOUT
THE AUTHOR

CHRIS WARK is an author, speaker, patient advocate and wellness crusader. He was diagnosed with stage III colon cancer in 2003 at 26 years old. He had surgery, but instead of chemotherapy, he used nutrition and natural therapies to heal himself. Chris has made many appearances on radio and television and was featured in the award-winning documentary film *The C Word*. Chris inspires countless people to take control of their health and reverse disease with a radical transformation of diet and lifestyle. www.chrisbeatcancer.com

HAY HOUSE

Look within

Join the conversation about latest products,
events, exclusive offers and more.

f Hay House

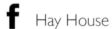 @HayHouseUK

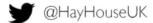 @hayhouseuk

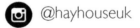 healyourlife.com

We'd love to hear from you!